the lowdown on
facelifts
and other **wrinkle**
remedies

**For Eden, whose blue eyes and bright smile
are the real beauty in my life**

First published in 2001 by
Quadrille Publishing Limited
Alhambra House
27-31 Charing Cross Road
London WC2H 0LS

This edition first published in 2002

Editorial Director Jane O'Shea
Art Director Mary Evans
Editor Clare Hill
Designer Jim Smith
Production Julie Hadingham

Illustrations Bridget Bodoano

Cataloguing in Publication Data: a catalogue record for this book
is available from the British Library.

ISBN 1 903845 80 7
Printed and bound by Mackays of Chatham, England.

the lowdown on facelifts and other wrinkle remedies

Wendy Lewis

Quadrille

contents

foreword – Alan Matarasso, MD FACS

Plastic surgery represents the interface between art and science. It is neither an exact science nor a magical art. The goal of well-performed cosmetic plastic surgery is to help you look as good as your anatomy and skin texture will allow. The facelift remains the gold standard of facial rejuvenation techniques and the most rewarding for both the plastic surgeon and the patient. Surgery will improve contour (what is loose), and non-surgical procedures such as creams or chemicals will enhance the skin's texture (lines, crow's feet, creases, and so forth). In each case, choosing one method and excluding the others may only address some of your concerns. The modern approach to correcting the signs of ageing is with less invasive and more limited procedures that produce a rejuvenating effect but let you return to your life more rapidly, with state-of-the-art skin preparations, fillers, resurfacing techniques and BOTOX injections used to treat expression lines.

Some of the factors influencing the final outcome of a facelift are not entirely under the control of either the surgeon or the patient. How any one patient will heal is not always predictable. Subsequently, the surgical results of facial, eyelid and brow surgery will vary between patients and are determined by numerous factors. These include the physical condition of the face (its intrinsic anatomy, including the underlying bone or dental structure), the thickness and quality of the skin (particularly its degree of sun damage), the depth and type of wrinkles, your hormonal and weight fluctuations, as well as heredity and other factors. If you expect a transforming miracle from cosmetic surgery, you will unquestionably be disappointed.

It is not possible to make someone who is 50 look 25 again. While this may seem obvious, misconceptions and misinformation can make one believe that the clock can be turned back in this fashion; it cannot. We cannot attempt to erase every fine line or tighten every millimetre of loose skin without the risk of pulling the skin and tissues too tight. This is especially true on the neck, where thinned skin will only respond so much to surgical alteration. The result of too much tension is distorted skin, widened scars, elevated hairlines, and the 'wind tunnel' look – all tell-tale signs of surgery. Early application of skincare products can improve and delay the onset of ageing, especially in difficult areas such as the neck.

Facial rejuvenation surgery can reset time but it cannot stop its progress. The results of surgery will not suddenly 'fall down', but they will succumb to time, gravity and the ageing process. How soon you will need another lift is highly individualized. In general, face and neck lifting, which is the improvement of the jowls along the jaw line and the loose skin of the neck, may need to be redone in 5 to 10 years, depending on your age at the time of your operation and how you maintain yourself. Smoking, alcohol intake, weight fluctuations and sun exposure will significantly shorten the life of your facelift. Some patients age more rapidly than others so another lift may be needed or desired sooner. Others may opt for non-surgical 'maintenance' techniques instead of further surgery down the line. Operations to correct lower eyelid bags or heaviness of the upper eyelids usually last longer than facial surgery and are considered 'semi-permanent'. In most instances, the pouches beneath the lower lids do not recur, but as you grow older, the skin becomes looser and fine lines reappear and deepen. Wrinkles around the eyelids and crows feet can be treated with lasers, chemical peels or BOTOX injections.

You can always expect to look better after surgery. However, the younger you are and the less damaged your skin is, the better a result you can expect – and the longer it will last. The older you are and the more visible the signs of ageing in your face and neck, the shorter duration your facelift will have. There is no one ideal rejuvenation technique for all faces. The most effective facelift is one that includes tightening the facial skin and muscles below, as well as sculpting the fat for the best aesthetic contour. When I began in private practice we had one procedure, but now we have the tools to tailor each operation to the individual. The future is limited only by our sense of innovation, coupled with sound medical and surgical judgment.

Alan Matarasso is a leading aesthetic plastic surgeon. He is a member of the American Society of Plastic Surgeons and the American Society for Aesthetic Plastic Surgery.

introduction

– confessions of a cosmetic surgery consultant

I've spent the better part of the past two decades in the constantly evolving world of cosmetic surgery and have seen it from all vantage points. I worked for two aesthetic plastic surgeons in New York City for a total of twelve years, and was a patient several times. I have also had the good fortune to work closely with clients as an independent consultant both in the United States and in the UK. For many of my years in this field, I have recommended procedures, treatments and products to 'other' women considerably older than myself. Turning 40 changed that for me, and I became an eager listener and disciple of what I have learned along the way.

My earliest introduction to plastic surgery (it wasn't called cosmetic surgery back then) was the day I went for a job at the fashionable upper eastside townhouse of a renowned plastic surgeon in the summer of 1982. I knew virtually nothing about cosmetic surgery, except that 'deviated septum' really meant 'nose job', and that Raquel Welch's breasts were probably too perfect to be real.

Back then, women who were having plastic surgery made every attempt to hide the fact that they had had it done. Secret trap door entrances to clinics and long, mysterious absences after their facelifts were the norm. Regrettably, their surgeons didn't always follow suit. Techniques were such that lifted faces and cheeks injected with liquid silicone were painfully obvious to all. Phenol peels were stylish then, and you could often catch a glimpse of yourself in the shiny reflection of peeled foreheads. Women wanted their noses to look like the sinewy sculpted tip of model Katherine Graham's, as featured in Estée Lauder advertisements for several years. Celebrities rarely disclosed more than good genes and meditation, with the exception of Phyllis Diller and Joan Rivers, who turned their cosmetic surgery adventures into comedy. In the UK, no one admitted to anything, not even covering up the grey, and even today the rule of thumb remains 'deny, deny, deny'.

Fifteen years ago, a woman who was considering cosmetic surgery would confide in a close girlfriend whom she suspected was no stranger to the knife, and went to the same surgeon. If she was given a few names, she may have gone to see two of them, and ultimately chose the one she liked best. If she did see more than one doctor, it was likely that she got the identical recommendations from all of them. The consultation of yester-year typically lasted a quarter of an hour, and the total number of procedures routinely performed by plastic surgeons numbered no more than a dozen. When the same woman wanted a second go at it, she generally went back to the same surgeon, unless of course she was unhappy with her first procedure. If she wasn't pleased, she found a new doctor, tried one on the other coast, or swore off surgery altogether. The range of fees was far more narrow back then, and prices were considerably lower. Fewer people were having cosmetic surgery, and fewer procedures were being done at the same time. There were also a lot fewer doctors doing cosmetic surgery in the early 1980s, and the field was limited to plastic surgeons only. Finally, the typical cosmetic patient of fifteen years ago was also more likely to write a cheque to pay for her operation outright, without the benefit of a credit card or 36-month financing plans.

Today it is very different. We are experiencing an explosion of the information age that has resulted in an overload of contradictory and unreliable information masquerading as facts and science. We don't know whom or what to believe any more. The credibility of the beauty consultant at the makeup counter, once considered the bastion of advice on skincare and cosmetics, has been undermined. We no longer take product or treatment recommendations at face value without questioning economic incentives and motives. The smorgasbord of choices available today to prolong beauty and youth is overwhelming to most of us, no matter where you call home. As a result, women are caught in a quagmire of uncertainty.

In the United States, most people considering cosmetic procedures will see several surgeons first for consultations. The more surgeons they see, the more confused they become. They may see two plastic surgeons, one facial plastic surgeon and a dermatologist, even though they often don't have a clear understanding of the differences in training and credentials between the professions. Also, it is not unusual to get conflicting opinions from many of the surgeons they consult. They are more willing to travel to have cosmetic procedures for many reasons, including price, and choose surgeons based on advertisements, the latest technology, articles in women's magazines, and the Internet. Today's patients compare notes, check out fees, ask friends and other specialists for referrals, read books, and do not hide the fact that they shop around. They are better informed, more knowledgeable about the specifics of procedures and techniques, and often know what they want before they ever get to a doctor's office.

The reverse phenomenon is true in the UK. British women, it seems, are generally of a different mindset. The American preoccupation with feeling and looking younger is exporting its influence across The Pond. The stigma of cosmetic treatments and procedures is slowly being lifted in the UK and no longer carries the great fear and loathing it once did. However, now that women are finally allowing themselves the luxury of exploring and experimenting with beauty enhancements and anti-ageing therapies, they are curiously lost and often find that they have nowhere to turn for expert advice.

If you are thinking about having something done to your wrinkles or your saggy neck, you will have little information to consider unless you are fortunate enough to have a close friend who is willing to guide you. The Internet will ultimately put the UK woman on a level playing field with her US counterpart, but it will take time. Until then, it seems to me that women in the UK are at a supreme disadvantage by not having access to the vital information required to make informed decisions.

My interest in the UK began quite accidentally in October of 1997, just four months after I had started my beauty consultancy. I was hosting an event entitled, 'Am I Ready For A Facelift?' featuring three well-known plastic surgeons on the panel. Unbeknownst to any of the guests or speakers (myself included), a member of the audience was the New York correspondent for the London Evening Standard, who was so fascinated that she wrote up a full page article about it for the paper. The article appeared in Monday's evening edition, and my line first started ringing in the wee hours of Tuesday morning. After the first caller's refrain, 'we really need someone like you over here', I knew that London was softly beckoning me.

And therein lies the heart of this book's mission. It is a personal approach to sorting through some of the hope from the hype, and a reflection of the message I deliver to my private clients. The mantra they hear from me is simply, DO YOUR HOMEWORK. I give them the lowdown on supposedly 'new' techniques, teach them where to get solid information, what questions to ask, what to watch out for, when to walk away, and how to keep it all in perspective. If they know what to expect, they are less likely to be disappointed with the results of whatever wrinkle remedies they choose for themselves.

We are witnessing a global shift of power from the sellers to the buyers. For an educated consumer, it is truly a buyer's market. I would rather be in my 40s today than at any other time in history.

Wendy Lewis

1

ageing gracefully is for cabernet

Growing old might not seem all that bad, but looking old is definitely the pits. Inevitably, somewhere in your fourth decade, you begin to spot the earliest signs of visible ageing creeping up on you. Even if you think you're prepared, once those signs appear, it can be a real shock. The trigger event could be the first grey hair you pluck out, or when the third person of the day asks whether you got enough sleep last night. The subtleties are there. For me, it was when I received an envelope of photos taken at an event I had hosted. Eden, my daughter (like all little girls, she thinks her mother is beautiful), exclaimed, 'Those pictures didn't come out so good. Your face looks fuzzy.' She was innocently referring to the jowling and puffiness that are telltale signs of a gravitational descent that started in that decade or so between 30 and 40.

Once you have turned that corner, the young appearance you took for granted in your 20s now takes hard work. The 'less is more' philosophy of makeup, skin care and fashion just won't cut it any more. The older you get, the more you need to look good – and that means using more day and night creams with more active ingredients and taking more care and attention over the details. This makes you definitely high maintenance. At this age, when you're just too weary to give your skin a good cleansing before you flop into bed, you'll pay for it in the morning. You need consistently better makeup tools and skills to create the natural 'no-makeup' look. Product descriptions such as 'sheer', 'light' and 'purifying' lose their appeal and are quickly replaced by the anticipation of the virtues of 'age-defying', 'time release' and 'rejuvenating'. I now set my alarm 15 minutes earlier just to give myself time to complete the arduous process of putting myself together. I start with an all-day intensive moisturizer with a high SPF, followed by something loosely referred to as 'maximum coverage', and a bronzing powder to simulate the rosy glow I no longer have as I avoid all contact with natural light. I never leave home without the security of my emergency makeup case, and am now adept at touching up lip-liner and dabbing on concealer with the aid of a taxi mirror.

I have no 8x power magnifying mirrors in my bathroom any more – I threw them out when I hit 35. If others can't see it with the naked eye, I don't have time to worry about it. (It has crossed my mind, however, now that laser vision correction is giving the world perfect vision, that there's no telling exactly what the naked eye can see any more.) Like most of the women I counsel, I peer in the mirror just long enough to make sure I don't have oregano in my teeth or mascara smudges, but rarely do I linger longer. My Filofax is cluttered with dates for 'beauty fixes' such as the frown eliminator BOTOX, the line plumper collagen, numerous facial treatments and high maintenance haircare. With what I've spent to be blonde, I could have bought a holiday home on the Côte d'Azure by now.

Just this year I stood helplessly by, watching the corners of my mouth pointing south and my fine lines deepening into folds. Now I'm inching my way to lifting something but I'm not sure what yet or in what order. The irony is that although I know the process started some time ago, it feels like it happened in just a fortnight.

stopping the clock – or slowing it down

Ageing is inevitable, but looking older than you have to is your choice – and not a very popular one. Stopping the clock may seem more desirable than merely slowing the tempo, but the best we can do for now is to turn back the clock a little, and start the meter running again from that point. One thing is for certain: whatever you do and whenever you do it, your face will be better off because you did it, rather than if you hadn't, or if you had waited longer.

I have come to the realization that the true life cycle of a woman can be divided into three distinct stages. First, there are the 'Adorable' years: the 21 to 32-ish range when you are cute enough to get away with almost anything. These years are generous and forgiving – you can abuse your body and still look fresh as a daisy. Next come the 'Seductive' years: the 30-something to 45-ish era. During this period we become too old to be young but too young to be middle-aged. This is when we experience the first signs of ageing. The next phase is the 'Maintenance Zone', which is a holding pattern of sorts. It begins sometime during the Seductive decade and should ideally overlap with the Maintenance years. The Maintenance phase used to begin much later in life but we start earlier now, in keeping with the philosophy that it's never too soon to start. It's never too late to start either, but clearly the sooner the better. A well-planned and early segue into the Maintenance zone can extend the half-life of the Seductive period considerably.

After the passing of the Maintenance zone, we approach the time when we're old enough not to give a hoot about any of this any more and it's better to simply lose count of the years.

The goal for modern and forward-thinking women is to prolong each of these ages for as long as possible. The longer we can extend the 'Adorable' years, and cling to our 'Seductive' years, the less time we will have left for the 'Lost' years.

These truisms, of course, do not apply to men. Although there have been sightings of males buying sun creams and designer shaving gels, as well as patronizing Mayfair salons for an infrequent facial or

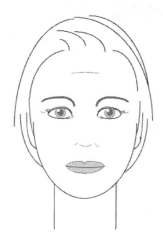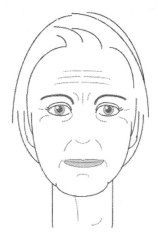

Seductive years   **Maintenance years**

massage, the male gender will never catch up. The Wrinkle Report IV, conducted by Harris Interactive in 1999 on behalf of Ortho Dermatological, determined that women spend an average of 19 minutes a day on their facial appearance. By comparison, men spend about 11 minutes, probably most of them devoted to admiring themselves in the bathroom mirror.

I've long been fascinated by exactly how many beauty products it takes to get through a typical day in the life of a real woman. I have surveyed several girlfriends on both sides of The Pond on this critical issue and discovered that few of us have actually taken the time to do the sums. However, you might be surprised to learn that 10 products wouldn't get most of us through to lunchtime. I came up with 29 products (see A day in the life of a well-groomed woman, overleaf) on average, and I'm not talking about false eyelashes and three kinds of hair mousses. That number varies seasonally and may drop sharply in the summer when whatever you put on your face slides off in a minute and a half anyway. In the winter, the total often climbs dangerously close to my actual chronological age. If you don't believe me, do your own count and you'll see that you're probably not far off.

A day in the life of a well-groomed woman

For basic maintenance, a well-groomed woman might use the following products during a typical day. All products such as toothpaste and lipstick that are used more than once a day have only been counted once. Other products, such as shaving foam for grooming underarms and legs, have not been included.

In the morning

AT THE BASIN
1) Toothpaste

IN THE SHOWER
2) Shower gel
3) Shampoo
4) Conditioner

AFTER THE SHOWER
5) Body lotion
6) Deodorant
7) Talcum powder
8) Hair styling mousse
9) Eye cream
10) Daytime face moisturizer
11) Sunscreen

AT THE BATHROOM MIRROR
12) Concealer
13) Foundation
14) Powder
15) Eyeshadow
16) Eyebrow pencil
17) Mascara
18) Blusher
19) Lipstick
20) Lip-liner
21) Perfume

At bedtime

22) Eye makeup remover
23) Cleanser
24) Toner
25) Night cream
26) Eye cream
27) Body lotion
28) Hand cream

Despite the wealth of scientific advances that have been made to allow us to experience the surgical restoration of facial youth, you have to play your part, too. The better the condition of your skin and underlying tissues, the more you can expect from your cosmetic surgeon. If you've spent years in the sun tempting fate, and most of your adult years ignoring the value of deep exfoliation, no amount of beauty treatments or weekends at a health farm can do what a lifetime of good grooming and lifestyle choices could have done in the first place. You've got to give the doctors something to work with. According to Dr Fritz Barton, Past President of the American Society of Aesthetic Plastic Surgery, 'The quality of the skin is as important to plastic surgeons as the quantity of the skin.' Plastic surgeons like to operate on good skin. They also like to operate on healthy, attractive and well-maintained women. It makes their job easier, and they get infinitely better surgical results with fewer healing problems.

wrinkle futures – outsmarting your genes

One of the best things you can give your cosmetic surgeon to work with is a good gene pool. Dr Sheldon Pinnell, Professor of Dermatology at Duke University, and better known as the 'Vitamin C Guru', says that, 'If you want to know how you will age, look at your parents.' I've never looked at my mother the same way since. Despite the miracles of modern science, your parents still largely predetermine your pattern of ageing. The blessing of being born with good genes helps, but heredity is one of those niggling things you have absolutely no control over. It's just the luck of the draw. This does not mean that if your mother started to shrivel earlier rather than later, your fate is permanently sealed. It should be looked upon rather as an indicator that you would be wise to pay special attention during the Adorable years previously referred to, and take all the necessary precautions.

My grandmother had roots in a little town in Northern Italy called Massa Carrara, named after the marble quarries found there. As a girl, her mother, like most Mediterranean women during the early 1900s, fed her a tablespoon of pure virgin olive oil every day. She continued this ritual well into her 70s, and Grandma Julia had beautiful ivory skin up until the day she died – and the suitors to prove it. I am proud to say that I inherited her spectacular genes for good skin (along with her propensity for thighs the size of Montana). One of the supreme ironies in genetics is that you have to take the bad with the good. We can't pick the ones we want and throw the others back, although that is exactly where the science of genetic engineering is clearly going.

Along with genes that can produce clear skin, good bones are also inherited. High cheekbones, sturdy chins and defined jawlines are just some of those things that, like long legs, get passed down from generation to generation. How fast your facial tissues droop is determined at least in part by how much bony support the cheeks, chin and jaw provide. Chins that already recede will recede more as the years go by. This will accentuate changes in the neck caused by the loss of facial fat and bone density. The trouble with necks is that they have nowhere to go but down. The less you have to hold them up, the droopier they will get. The neck is one of the early places where ageing changes are visible, and it is also the area of the body that often makes you feel that you look older.

Good genes are always a welcome gift, but they do not guarantee great skin or beautiful bones, nor do they offer any assurance of protection from the preventable symptoms of ageing. By preventable I mean the external forces within your control, as opposed to ones you cannot control, like choosing your parents.

your lifestyle may be ageing you

Environmental and lifestyle factors have a big impact on the skin. The most rejuvenating product you can have in your medicine cabinet is sun block. Golf, tennis, sailing, riding, gardening, a home beside the sea are just some of the benefits of living the good life. But, unless you practise diligent sun protection, they can also contribute to prematurely aged and wrinkled skin, even when the sun isn't shining.

Once upon a time the only thing a woman had to know about her skin was whether it was dry, normal or oily. Then along came the next generation of categories for those who weren't sure; normal/dry and normal/oily. Determining skin types today has taken on a whole new dimension. 'Oily' has become the new 'dry' skin. Also, squillions of people were walking around blushing and looking embarrassed for centuries before it was determined that they actually had rosacea, a skin condition characterized by red, flushed facial skin. One might conclude that prior to the 1990s chronic skin conditions commonly known as 'rosacea' and 'acne vulgaris' were obscure mutations visited upon a select few teenagers as punishment for poor school records and spending too much time watching videos. The truth is that ever since God made hormones, there were pimples.

Case history

Caitlin Graham, aged 36, was obsessed with the condition of her skin. Her continuous eruptions were the cause of much embarrassment and she was keen to do, buy or use anything to make them go away.

After some inquiry, Caitlin described the facial massage treatments she was having on a weekly basis for the past year and the creams she was given to use in between. When asked if her skin looked better now than when she first began the treatments, she replied with a sheepish 'not really'. In her zeal to improve her skin, Caitlin had fallen prey to an unscrupulous salon operator who had her hooked on the wrong treatment at the cost of several hundred pounds a month. One visit to a consultant dermatologist set her right. He gave her a course of retinoids and benzoyl peroxide and now Caitlin is spot-free.

As with other difficult personal life events such as divorce, depression and the onset of menopause, spots rarely used to be discussed in an open forum. Most women would never dream of admitting in public to getting an occasional blemish. Spots were a rite of passage solely experienced during adolescence, up there with razor burn on the legs, bad haircuts and holes pierced in weird places. You were expected to simply light a candle and say a prayer, cover the conspicuous blemish with mounds of orange-tinted benzoyl-peroxide lotions, and hope against sense and reason for it to go before your big night out. Today, spotty breakouts have joined the ever-growing list of common-or-garden afflictions in the life of the modern woman, along with 'perimenopause' and 'feminine dryness'.

One explanation offered for the over-population of the skincare market with products targeting 'oily' and 'acne prone' skin types, is stress. Along with the ravaging effects of time and harmful free radicals in the environment, stress can really throw your beauty goals off track. There is no doubt about it; we live in stressful times. The majority of women work full-time plus, sometimes having 2 or 3 jobs on the go if you consider taking care of tots and tykes, husband and boyfriends, ageing parents and the home.

I know what stress does to me. On the eve of a deadline, slumped over my Victorian walnut desk chair with my swollen wrist joints perched on the keyboard, there is at least one broken nail I haven't had time to file and a combination of Tipp-Ex and black ink marks on my hands. My hair is piled on my head and clamped in place in a feeble attempt to camouflage the roots, a hoard of empty Evian bottles lie at my feet, and there is that crowding thing going on around my deepened eye sockets. My skin feels like I should dive face first into the 16-ounce tub of Crème de la Mer to re-hydrate it back to life. Let's just say I look vaguely like a distant cousin to the blonde on the book cover and leave it at that.

If you've got stress, it is an indicator that you lead a busy life. You've got places to go, people to see and plenty of things to do. You carry your mobile close by because people always need to reach you to make important decisions affecting national security. Every woman thinks she is very busy, including those who have virtually nothing to do all day. If you are accustomed to having three things to do in a day, adding a fourth would indeed cause you to be very busy, compared to your usual lifestyle, although I'm not quite sure that a frown-lifting BOTOX shot counts as one more thing. Everything is relative.

Stress deprives you of your nightly beauty sleep, causing shadows, dark circles and puffiness around the eyes, as well as headaches. It causes non-smokers to smoke, and smokers to smoke like chimneys. It drives teetotallers to sip a pungent yet alluring Chardonnay, and wine drinkers to hit the malt hard. Smoking, being around smokers, and drinking alcohol daily can turn a pretty 35 year old into a wrinkled hag faster than you can say 'FACELIFT'.

The science of skin – what ages it faster
- Drinking alcohol (beer, wine, cocktails, spirits, liqueurs)
- Smoking (cigarettes, cigars, pipes – they all count)
- Sun exposure (even when the sun isn't shining)
- Wind burn (ahoy sailors and skiers)
- High stress (at work, at home, at play)
- Lack of sleep (clubbing, late nights, restlessness, insomnia)
- Fad dieting (fat-free, carb-free & nutrient-free)
- Dehydration (not enough water intake – Diet Coke doesn't count)

too young to look old – what age
to start thinking about ageing

Not surprisingly, women are starting to think about wrinkles much earlier in chronological terms than in previous generations. It would have been considered a sure sign of Obsessive Compulsive Disorder for a 20-something female to start shopping for wrinkle creams in our mothers' era. We are experiencing a shift in the anti-ageing category to include everyone from over the age of 21. The curve is starting to bend from 'approaching 40' to 'mid-30s' and dropping closer to just plain '30'.

It's all a matter of degree. The diligent and thin-skinned among us aren't willing to take any chances and begin fretting and hanging around beauty counters at around the age of 30. The braver, perpetual optimists among us will dismiss worrying about wrinkles as nothing more than a foolish pastime of the idle and shallow. It will just take them a little longer to join the rest of us in the Cosmetics Hall of our local department store.

Estée Lauder introduced an eye product appropriately titled Unline Total Eyecare. The provocative tag line that follows should hit home with every woman who has ever witnessed the footprint of a crow's line: *Have you seen your first line?* Few among the female gender would respond with anything other than the affirmative. The mere suggestion of the phrase instils a sense of urgent panic in any woman, and we duly respond as dogs to Pavlov. Without delay, we are compelled to check in the closest mirror to be sure. Until you actually cross the threshold of discovering that first line, your greatest concerns are controlling occasional breakouts of spots and keeping up with the season's hot nail varnish colour.

Estée Lauder's marketing question of the day is '*Am I too young to start using an eye cream?*' The answer, says Lauder, is a resounding NO, thereby insuring a steady flow of the next generation of advanced treatment buyers – the 30 year olds.

undoing the damage

The goal of anti-ageing technology is a no-holds-barred attack to undo the damage you did in your 20s, when you thought your skin would look young forever. The earlier you start to pay attention to your complexion and stop taking it for granted, the better prepared you'll be for the decades to follow. We have access to technology that can actually reverse the visible signs of damage and it can make a real difference in the quality of your skin. The key is to determine the best combination for you.

There are no broad brushstrokes that can convey the variability of ageing. It is not a uniform experience, but rather a very personal phenomenon. The numerous factors that affect the rate and degree to which your skin will show signs of ageing make it virtually impossible to compare your skin condition to that of your contemporaries. It is also hard to take a step back and remain objective. Just because your sister-in-law's skin looks great, does not necessarily mean you should run out and buy what she is using. Every woman's skin responds differently – and has different needs at different stages.

I was peacefully wending my way through the aisles at Boot's one evening and overheard a conversation brewing at the counter. A young woman was trying to pick a foundation, as the one she had been using was too dry. She said she had slightly oily skin, and wanted something in between her last one and a true moisturizing formula that she was afraid might give her spots. The beauty adviser behind the counter was clearly stumped, so the woman guarding the cash register chimed in to help make the sale. A customer browsing nearby also felt moved to offer advice and piped up, 'Whatever formula you choose, you will need a moisturizer'. Her personal favourite was Lancôme's Primordiale, although she was about 10 years older than the girl shopping for foundation. The guardian of the cash register confirmed that Primordiale was indeed brilliant, but she was at least 10 years and multiple wrinkles older than anyone else in the shop. The beauty adviser then suggested that a tinted moisturizer might be good, although they were out of stock. I peered over the jungle of hair mousses in my aisle as the frustration mounting in the customer's face began to create a marked crease between her brows that would necessitate early intervention with BOTOX. She stood perfectly still as everyone observed a moment of pensive silence. Her overactive forehead muscles contracted vigorously as she considered the options laid before her. She then turned quietly and exited the shop.

In this age of beauty retailers and e-tailers, personalized service seems to be disappearing rapidly. The advice you get is often no more than a reasonable guess, and usually without confirmation from any other source. Although I admit to being a great devotee of some of the most luxurious skincare products on the market, like most women I mix-and-match expensive speciality products with great bargains from pharmacy and high street discount shops, and I also throw in a little bit of everything in between. Whether your budget is £10 or £100 for each product, you can have your pick of a great assortment in every price range and formula your heart desires. Some of my favourites suitable for a wide range of ages in all price categories are listed throughout the chapters that follow.

Skin products that you buy over-the-counter can make good skin look and feel better, but if you want to erase the signs of sun damage that rest deeper than the skin's surface you'll need to shop for a 'cosmeceutical' product (a range of 'active' products that slot in somewhere between the Lancôme counter and the cosmetic surgeon's office). Until very recently, cosmeceuticals had the disadvantage of coming in generic brown medicine bottles and white plastic jars, without a whiff of fragrance or a scintilla of elegance. The psychological and emotional side to a woman's choice in wrinkle remedies cannot be overlooked.

There is a phenomenon that exists within the process of selecting skincare: a woman's willingness to commit to products devoid of all traces of elegance is directly correlated to how bad her skin looks. Although I confess to lacking the requisite hard data to actually prove this theory beyond a reasonable doubt, I firmly believe it to be true. A woman with good to excellent skin may try the latest, most touted anti-ageing skin treatments once, but she is far less likely to finish the jar or purchase it again if it isn't pleasurable to use. The fact remains that no matter how performance-based and ingredient-infused the anti-ageing formula is, if a woman doesn't like the way it feels, smells and wears, she isn't going to use it for long.

4 steps to age defiance
- **Prevention** – prevent early environmental damage (wear a sunscreen, even when the sun is hiding)
- **Protection** – protect from future damage (wear a sunscreen and a moisturizer)
- **Reversal** – reverse existing damage (wear a sunscreen and a moisturizer, and use anti-ageing products)
- **Maintenance** – keep it all up (do it every day)

the big picture – no one single thing
can prevent premature ageing

Retarding the ageing process is not a one-shot deal. You can't have a few skin peels, slap on some fancily packaged serum, down a few anti-oxidants and call it a day. It requires a consistent and integrated programme of a little of this with a lot of that and absolutely none of the other. If you use sun cream with a high sun protection factor (SPF) and UVA/UVB protection (see overleaf), but you smoke a pack of Gitanes every day, one just about cancels the other out. Similarly, if you go riding three times a week but forget to wear sun protection or a floppy hat with a brim, what little sun there is could be doing more to make you look older than all that aerobic exercise is doing to keep you young.

To say that we live in an information age is a vast understatement. I suppose it is better to have too much information than too little. The former challenges your brain to process the tools it needs to make intelligent decisions, while the latter keeps you perpetually in the dark. Motivation is the distinguishing factor. Every woman places a different emphasis on the issues that affect her decision-making. For example, the knowledge that nicotine will cause brown stains on your glistening porcelain veneers may not be enough to move you to stop smoking. However, when your cosmetic surgeon tells you he won't pull you as tightly as you need because you're a smoker, you may finally have the impetus you needed to try Nicorette. If you love pruning your rose garden but refuse to wear more than an SPF8 because you like the way you look with a light tan, the solution is not to give up your passion for roses. You can invest in a floppy hat and a trunk of Clarins Self-Tanning Face Lotion Very High Protection without risking the revenge of the free radicals.

Behaviour modification is like marriage – it's all a matter of compromise. You give up something that is less important to you than something else, or make substitutions as you go along.

sunscreen update

If the Surgeon General said smoking causes wrinkles, women wouldn't smoke.

Arlene Dahl, actress

If you want peachy skin throughout life, wear sunscreen at all times when you are outside – even if the sun isn't shining. The damage to skin is caused by the sun's ultraviolet A (UVA) and ultraviolet B (UVB) rays. UVA rays are long-wave solar rays that penetrate the skin more deeply and are considered the biggest cause of wrinkling and changes in the texture of your skin. UVB rays are short-wave solar rays that are more potent than UVA in causing sunburn, and are the chief culprit for the development of skin cancer. Look out for sun protection factor (SPF) ratings on the sunscreen packaging and choose a broad-spectrum product that deflects both UVA and UVB rays, like those containing:

Parsol 1789
Titanium Dioxide
Micronized Zinc

The packaging will tell you what sort of SPF the product provides:

Minimum protection (SPF 2–12)
Moderate protection (SPF 12–30)
High protection (SPF 30 plus)

According to the British Association of Dermatology, high factor sunblock creams (Factor 15 or higher) will help prevent darkening of the skin in response to sunshine and, in the long run, reduce the 'ageing' changes, which the sun produces over a lifetime. The Association warns against intermittent intense exposure to ultraviolet radiation from sunlight, especially during the middle of the day (11am–3pm) in summer and when in sunny climates. This particularly applies to those with fair skin who burn easily. The Association does not advocate total sun avoidance, but it endorses the importance of reducing sun exposure and preventing sunburn by the use of appropriate clothing, shade, sunscreens and the avoidance of peak hours of sunshine.

type casting

Understanding your basic skin type can reveal how your skin might age, and how you can best prevent premature environmental damage. Dermatologists classify skin types according to the skin's tendency to sunburn, as follows:

Type	Complexion type	Extent of sun damage
Type I	Very pale: always burns, never tans	High
Type II	Fair skin and hair: burns easily, tans minimally	High
Type III	Slightly darker skin: burns sometimes, tans gradually	High to moderate
Type IV	Mediterranean: burns rarely, tans easily	Moderate
Type V	Asian/Arabic: burns rarely, always tans	Moderate to low
Type VI	Afro-Caribbean: never burns, always tans deeply	Low

(SOURCE: Ortho Division of Janssen-Cilag Ltd)

The more pigmentation (melanin) you have in your skin, the darker your skin colour. Melanin provides natural sun protection, which can prolong the appearance of visible signs of ageing. Light-skinned patients (Northern European) will start to see evidence of photo-ageing from age 29–35 and so require earlier intervention to protect the skin. Sun exposure causes structural damage to the layers of the skin and this causes a loss of the precious natural collagen in the skin that gives it its elasticity.

Darker skin types (Types IV, V and VI) develop fine lines much later because they are pigment-protected. As they tend to colour (pigment) before they burn, they are at risk of chronic hyperpigmentation or discolouration earlier in life. However, no matter what your skin type is, a minimum of SPF15 is recommended.

Darker skin types are not immune from the ravages of the sun, so the same rule applies. Very fair skin types (Types I and II) should use a higher SPF from the start.

After spending countless tax dollars to review the situation, the American Food and Drug Administration ruled that all non-SPF sun care products are required to say on the label that they do not contain sunscreen and that sun exposure causes premature ageing and skin cancer. This 'Sun Alert' message is akin to the warning on cigarette packs that smoking causes lung cancer, which even the tobacco growers have figured out by now. However, no one can really protect us from ourselves. Despite all good intentions, a skull and crossbones on the label would still not cause sales of Marlboro to drop significantly. Surely by now everyone must have heard the news that basking in the sun damages your skin and causes wrinkles, not to mention a deadly little thing called skin cancer.

Wrinkles, although unattractive and inconvenient, can be turned around, as you are about to find out. It is never too late to start reversing the ageing process.

a smorgasbord of wrinkle remedies

Beautiful skin is the best accessory

Katherine Betts

When we think of wrinkles, we think of skin – specifically the skin on the face, neck and around the eyelids. Ageing leaves its imprint on the complexion most dramatically because the skin in these areas is the thinnest and the most overexposed. The face is also the first thing other people see. The parts of the body below the neck have more time than the face to catch up with the ageing process. The delicate facial skin first starts to wrinkle, then crease and fold, and then it makes a quantum leap right over to sagging. That is simply a fact of life and a rite of passage.

One of the great fallacies about cosmetic surgery is that if you want to get rid of wrinkles, you need to go under the knife. This is not true. The way to treat wrinkles is generally not with surgery, as this is almost never the logical first step. The end result of a facelift that has been carried out on old-looking, wrinkled and dry skin is a lifted face with tighter old-looking, wrinkled and dry skin. Surgical intervention will only redrape the crêpey skin of the face and neck, which will go quite far to reduce your double chins and turkey neck, but you will still have your wrinkles.

The place to start is with brilliant skincare, followed by or in tandem with a combination of non-surgical treatments, such as collagen and/or BOTOX, and laser skin treatment. Surgery should only happen when the time is right. Having had a front row seat in cosmetic surgery and dermatology for well over two decades, Christina Carlino, Chief Executive Officer of Philosophy, explains, 'You have to take baby steps, beginning with a comprehensive skin rejuvenation programme that can rehabilitate your skin from scalp to toe.' Although nothing to date will produce the tightening and rejuvenating results of a facelift operation, maintenance will help you forestall the need for such invasive measures until later.

Not every woman will have a facelift in her lifetime, but with today's menu of non-surgical alternatives and potent topical products that can work very well, there is literally something for every face and every budget. Consider these examples:

TYPE I – The Beginner

The typical woman I see in London is 53 years old but looks 63. She doesn't colour the grey in her hair and considers a rosy glow from sitting in her garden to be a sure sign of good health. She cares for her skin by washing with Imperial Leather soap and using a dab of Nivea occasionally when her skin feels dry. And that is it. She has prematurely aged fine and fair skin, superficial wrinkling and her husband of thirty years thinks 'she looks fine'. However, she feels that she's starting to look old. The only time she has ever seen a consultant dermatologist was for a burn on her hand.

TYPE II – The Shopper

In contrast, the typical woman who consults me in the New York area is aged anywhere from 35 to 65 and comes with a list of questions that reads like the Dead Sea Scrolls, complete with pages printed off the Internet and a variety of magazine clippings. She has a pretty good idea of what she needs and wants done and will move on, seeing various face specialists until she finds the 'best' doctor to trust her face to. She already sees a dermatologist for skin conditions such as psoriasis and suspicious moles, and also has the occasional collagen shot or laser peel. Expensive professionals regularly attend to her nails, hair and makeup.

TYPE III – The Trend Watcher

The other extreme is the client from the West Coast of the United States. Typically she is anywhere from 20-something to 50-something, and is no stranger to cosmetic work. She has friends who have used 'so and so' and done 'such and such'. She probably had her nose bobbed in high school and her eyes done early, several things injected or implanted into her lips to keep them perpetually swollen, and maybe breast implants and a little lipo, but that's all... Her face is permanently frozen from BOTOX overload and it's difficult to tell whether she is content or enraged at any given time. She drops the names of a handful of celebs whose work she thinks looks great and already knows who all the big-name cosmetic surgeons are.

Most women fall loosely into one of the above three categories, regardless of whether they live in Leeds or Los Angeles. There are some distinct geographic, cultural and philosophical differences, of course. According to Kathleen Walas, Group Vice President, Public Relations and Corporate Affairs at Avon, 'Our 2000 Avon Global Women's Survey revealed that while there are some regional differences in women's attitudes towards beauty and beauty products, ultimately women around the world share an unbelievable consistency in their attitudes. For example, the vast majority of women we polled – 85 per cent – agreed that outward appearance is an important part of defining who they are. Therefore, it is not surprising that most women (82 per cent) agree that beauty products are a necessity, not a luxury.'

If you aren't sure where you fall on this, make yourself a cup of tea, put your feet up and take our Multiple Choice Personal Assessment (page 188). Being female, we all have similar concerns about ageing, but to different degrees. The amount of funds and time you have and your tolerance for discomfort also factor into beauty decisions. However, treatment cosmetics and skincare are an absolute must always and, compared to other wrinkle remedies, they are good value.

hope in a jar, bottle, tube, dropper, pump, bar, etc – the marriage of cosmetics and pharmaceuticals

Anti-ageing formulations fall into three classifications: over-the-counter (cosmetics), non-prescription (cosmeceuticals), and prescription (drugs). There is a highly charged debate among dermatologists, cosmetics companies and regulatory agencies regarding the role of non-prescription strength active treatment products. The term 'cosmeceuticals' was coined by Professor Albert M. Kligman at the University of Pennsylvania during the late 1980s to cover an entirely new class of products that are a cross between a drug and a cosmetic. Since then, it has been broadened to encompass more than just a few fruit acids. Today's category of cosmeceuticals includes everything from retinoids (Vitamin A derivatives) to alpha hydroxy acids (AHAs) and beta hydroxy acids to Vitamins E, C, K, B-5 and other antioxidants, hyaluronic acid and high-tech ingredients known as 'bioactives' that have anti-ageing, slimming, skin lightening, firming and moisturizing effects. The ageing process is under increasingly intense scrutiny by the competitive scientific community. The race is on to develop formulas that target the symptoms of ageing that have been driving the growth in the global skincare market since the introduction of ingredients like retinol and AHAs in the early 1990s. So, is there life after alpha hydroxy acids and what will be the next generation of advanced ingredients?

An A to Z of anti-ageing skincare
Here is an easy guide to the high-tech side of skincare.

- **Alpha Hydroxy Acid (AHA)** – A group of acids derived from foods such as fruit and milk, the most common forms are Lactic Acid, Glycolic Acid, Pyruvic Acid, Tartaric Acid and Maleic Acid
- **Alpha Tocopherol** – Vitamin E, an oil-based antioxidant that moisturizes the skin by drawing its water content from the dermis to the epidermis
- **Alpha Lipoic Acid** – An antioxidant that fights free radicals in the fat and aqueous phases of cells
- **Antioxidant** – A substance designed to prevent a chemical reaction with oxygen, such as Vitamins C, E, A, grapeseed and green tea
- **Azelaic Acid** – A substance that has similar properties to retinoids (see Retinoeic Acid, below) and skin-lightening properties
- **Beta Hydroxy Acid (BHA)** - Acids that enhance cell renewal, such as salicylic, which is found naturally in willow bark.
- **Bioactives** –Substances that achieve cosmetic results by some degree of physiological action, for example, fruit acids
- **Ceramides** – Barrier-stabilizing components of the stratum corneum that restore the skin's natural condition
- **CoEnzyme Q10** – Ubiquinone, a fat-soluble antioxidant that is close to Vitamin E in structure
- **Hyaluronic acid** – A polysaccharide naturally found in the body's connective tissues; used as a moisturizing agent
- **Kojic Acid** – A natural skin-lightening agent derived from a Japanese mushroom
- **L-Ascorbic Acid** – The only form of Vitamin C the body can use to destroy harmful free radicals
- **Retinoeic Acid** – A Vitamin A-derived acid that speeds cell renewal and collagen production
- **Tazarotene** – A retinoid used for psoriasis and acne

There is a social trend among my own age group (aka 'Boomers') not to adopt the attitudes our parents had towards ageing. We are not part of the 'mature' market as it has been known, and refuse to embrace the terminology or inevitability of it. In our quest to delay the biological process of ageing, women over the age of 35 are making a significant impact on the face of the skincare market. In recent years, we have witnessed a surge in products featuring vitamins and botanical extracts cited for their ability to normalize, repair and protect skin from free radical damage, and these ingredients are showing up everywhere – including in toothpaste and pet food. Sweeping claims from manufacturers are making it harder to decipher what is valid from what is pure snake oil, but savvy beauty buyers are becoming increasingly more informed and are less likely to blindly accept manufacturers' claims. Today's serious skincare buyers are decidedly sceptical about the effectiveness of over-the-counter wrinkle creams without hard evidence to convince us to buy. Claims that promise 'a 67 per cent improvement in skin texture,' and 'up to 59 per cent reduction in fine wrinkles' attract a lot more excitement than the run-of-the-mill 'makes skin look and feel radiant and more youthful, blah, blah, blah…'.

If you want to rev up your skincare regimen a few notches, the best place to start is by adding one or more of the state-of-the-art anti-ageing basics. Systematic and informed use of tried and true rejuvenating ingredients can make a real difference in the quality of your skin. I do not mean you should scrap your collection of cleansers and toners right now, but rather that you should re-evaluate what you've got and see what's missing. The over-30s set should consider adding at least one 'active' product that provides the benefits of the best of today's advanced technologies. The key to defining 'active' is a product that contains an ingredient in a strong enough concentration which it delivers effectively into the skin to produce visible changes in texture and quality; in other words, a product that works beneath the skin's surface. The active ingredient should appear in the first three to five ingredients on the list. Retinoeic acid (Vitamin A), ascorbic acid (Vitamin C) and glycolic (alpha hydroxy) acids are widely considered to be the mainstays of an anti-ageing regimen, and the foundation from which to begin. There is a trend to develop increasingly more potent skincare treatment with higher levels of active ingredients in more elegant delivery systems, but with fewer of the side effects generally associated with high-tech formulations.

Most women have appallingly filthy skin. Good cleansing and frequent exfoliation are the secrets to young-looking skin.

Eve Lom, Facialist

Multi-purpose special treatments can be a dream come true for beauty junkies determined not to let any wrinkle get away. Some of these formulas can be likened to my colour printer/copier/ scanner/fax. Although it does it all, it does none of it well. It prints slowly, copies barely, scans in a low resolution and cannot fax at the same time as any of its other bells and whistles. For minimalists who want to have the fewest jars possible on their bathroom shelf, a formula with a pinch of C, a drop of A and E, and a tad of AHA sounds very attractive indeed. If you are the type that craves a kitchen sink sort of miracle cream, select one that has adequate protection from the evils of free radicals. Some cocktail formulas still do not contain sunscreen because adding sufficient levels of effective SPF can makes creams feel like mortar and wear like Polyfilla. Sunscreens (which absorb UV rays) and sunblocks (which deflect UV rays) should have a SPF15 (double that number if your skin is the colour of dairy products) and provide broad-spectrum protection, whether you live in Yorkshire or Sydney.

When your mother told you to eat your carrots, she was really on to something. Vitamin A, commonly found in yellow and orange vegetables such as carrots and peppers, has held its place in the realm of anti-ageing skincare ingredients. The impressive scientific data available on retinoeic acid (Retin-A and its cousins) for treating and preventing sun damage (photoageing) has inspired a generation of newcomers that offer some of the same properties without the flaking, redness and irritation. Retinoeic acid acts as a chemical peeling agent and helps the skin to renew itself more rapidly. According to Professor Nicholas Lowe, FRCP, FACP, 'Dermatologists of the 1940s and 1950s were right and Vitamin A does have special actions on the skin.

The therapeutic use of retinoids has had a revolutionary impact on a host of skin conditions including acne, rosacea and photo-ageing. There continues to be steady progress in developing newer retinoids, including formulas that are active against skin ageing (Tazarotene), and serious skin diseases such as lymphomas (Pan-Retin).'

Although many dermatologists would like to see the whole world on some form of Retin-A, it is not universally tolerated. There are those among us, myself included, who consider redness and irritation a sign from God that their active skincare is working. If there is no visible flaking, they remain unconvinced that it is really 'doing something'. Retinova is an emollient creamy formula of prescription strength Retin-A in a mineral oil base and is ideally suited for dry, ageing skin. It has the distinction of being the only wrinkle product approved by the American Food and Drug Administration in December 1995 for the treatment of wrinkles, and has been available in the UK since 1996. Retinova requires a prescription from a medical practitioner, and the price varies from £21–25 for a 20g tube.

Advice for Retinova use
- Use only at night on dry skin after cleansing
- Apply a pea-sized amount only
- Mild irritation, redness, dryness and peeling are common at first
- Use daily for 3–6 months to see results
- After 6–12 months, use 1–3 times weekly for maintenance
- Always use a broad-spectrum sunscreen SPF15 during the day

Retinova may be too creamy for you if your skin is oily or spot-prone, and your doctor may recommend Retin-A cream instead. If prescription grade retinoeic acid formulations are too irritating for you, try skipping a day, using it every two days, or applying it only to wrinkle-prone areas such as crow's feet, forehead lines and around the lips. You can also experiment with what dermatologists refer to as 'short contact therapy'. This means using a thin coat and washing it off after 10 minutes so that the drug penetrates enough but not too much. For the more timid among us, the next step down the ladder would be a retinol, which is an over-the-counter Vitamin A derivative that stimulates cell division and can, over time, reduce fine lines. Retinols come in every price range from department store or pharmacy brands at about £8, all the way up to prestige products that exceed the £100 mark. Although you won't see results as quickly with a retinol as with a consistent use of Retinova, some Vitamin A is better than none at all. The key is to start with a low concentration and work your way up to using the highest concentration that your skin can tolerate on a regular basis.

Plant enzymes are emerging as the next wave of hope in the battle against wrinkles. Kinerase from ICN Pharmaceuticals is one of the new kids on the block in anti-ageing technology. 'N6-Furfuryladenine', the chemical name for this plant growth factor, is being compared to retinoids for its effect on the skin. One of the properties of Furfuryladenine is that it is known to plump up the leaves of plants, and has a similar effect on human skin by causing the surface layer to retain water. Unlike traditional moisturizers, which temporarily add moisture to soften and plump the skin's texture, this plant enzyme enhances cell turnover.

The appeal of Kinerase is that it is non-irritating so almost anyone can use it and is available in both a lotion and a slightly richer cream formula. The same patented technology is available in the form of Kinetin from Osmotics, sold at beauty counters in certain department stores, and Skin Releaf with Kinetin from The Body Shop and Almay Kinetin. When I first heard of this technology, I confess that as a Manhattanite I have little access to the leaves of plants and could not make the connection. While browsing at Eli's, the Upper East Side's answer to Harrod's Food Hall, I paused momentarily at the greenery to feel a plant leaf en route to the salad bar. Kinerase does indeed leave skin leaf-soft and supple, but what remains to be seen is how it compares to the long-term benefits of retinoids. The good thing about this enzyme is that it has the flexibility of being easily incorporated into a regime of AHAs, Retinol or Vitamin C, or as an alternative if you prefer. It is also especially kind to recently peeled or lifted skin.

There is little doubt that cosmeceuticals are here to stay. This is not just some passing cosmetic fad that has peaked and is destined to go the way of wheatgrass juice. According to Phil Marchant, Oil of Olay's European Research and Development Manager, 'Our research has shown that women's concerns about their skin are far greater than just lines and wrinkles.' The properties now contained in cosmeceuticals and the extra benefits future formulas will contain are the next best thing to cosmetic surgery for skin rejuvenation. Cosmeceuticals have a definite role as a complement to surgery, rather than an alternative. No one can escape the skin changes that accompany age, but with a little help you can keep them under control.

7 signs of ageing world-wide

- the appearance of blotches and age spots (uneven pigment)
- skin texture (rough, scaly)
- skin tone (loose, slack)
- dryness (flaking, itching)
- visible pores (pores plugged with dirt that swell up)
- skin surface dullness (lack of vitality, poor colour)
- fine lines and wrinkles (eyes, around the mouth, forehead, neck)

(SOURCE: Oil of Olay Global Research)

Case history

Marie Cunningham, aged 53, journeys to central London for her collagen shots every other month. She has not been lifted yet, but has an exceptionally beautiful English complexion for a woman of her vintage. Marie swore me to secrecy when I inquired about her private wrinkle remedy. 'I use Retin-A 0.1% cream (the highest strength) all over my face every night, and plain Vaseline in the daytime,' she whispered, as if revealing the top-secret location of an arsenal of scud missiles. Although it clearly worked for Marie, I would be reluctant to suggest this regime to other clients for fear that they would use me for target practice for causing their pores to clog with petroleum jelly.

Active skincare - The A List

All these products contain some form of retinol, a derivative of Vitamin A. Retinols in over-the-counter products generally contain less than those available in cosmeceutical products, which are available at specialist outlets. Retinoids that are prescription-only have the highest concentration and must be used under the guidance of a medical professional.

- **COSMETIC** (over-the-counter)
  La Prairie Age Management Stimulus
  Christian Dior Phenomenon A
  Estée Lauder Diminish
  Guerlain Beautyssime A
  Erno Laszlo Retinol Reparative Therapy
  Lancôme Re-Surface
  Helena Rubinstein Power A
  Elizabeth Arden Millennium Energist
  RoC Retinol Pur Actif

- **SPECIALIST** (non-prescription)
  BioMedic Retinol
  Jan Marini Factor A
  Sothys Retinol
  MD Formulations Vit-A-Plus

- **PHARMACEUTICAL** (prescription-only)
  For ageing skin:
  Retinova 0.05% cream
  For acne:
  Retin-A cream (0.1%, 0.05%, 0.025%) or gel (0.025%, 0.01%)
  Differin Gel
  Roaccutane (Isotretinoin)
  Isotrex (topical Isotretinoin gel)
  For psoriasis:
  Zorax (topical Tazarotene)

turn over those cells

As we age, the process of cell turnover slows down along with our metabolism, reflexes and tolerance for stupidity, and we need a booster to stimulate the cycle after age 30. The art and science of exfoliation has become an integral part of a well-groomed woman's daily regime for healthy skin. It is commonly known that skin peels and regular exfoliation of dead cells can improve the immediate look of the skin, and instant gratification can have the greatest impact. Consistent exfoliation thins the thickened skin that piles up on the surface making your skin look dull, to produce an ongoing vitality in skin texture and quality. Pretty soon it will become acceptable to miss a social engagement because of it. The excuse of yesteryear, 'I can't make it tonight, I have to wash my hair', will shortly reinvent itself as 'Maybe next time, I have to exfoliate this evening.'

The tools of modern exfoliation run the gamut from substances squeezed out of a tube to mechanical devices. Abrasive sponges, loofahs and the flannels in your bathroom can all be used as exfoliants, as are the grainy formulas containing micro particles that are found in scrubs and soaps. AHAs are one of the most popular ingredients used for unclogging embedded cellular debris in the skin's pores and shedding the outermost layer of dead skin. If you stop using your AHAs, your skin will gradually revert to its normal, sluggish turnover rate. With continued use, AHA exfoliation has been shown to achieve a healthier appearance for a wide range of skin types and conditions including wrinkles, texture, tone, breakouts, blotches and age spots.

However, the current obsession with exfoliating is also responsible for the creation of an underclass of 'sensitive skin' sufferers. Layering ascorbic acid (Vitamin C) over retinoeic acid (Vitamin A) over glycolic acid will take its toll on our thinning, ageing skin. The result of self-treating wrinkles with potent chemicals and without the benefit of genuine expert advice is leading to a new strain of skin condition that is sure to find its way into dermatological literature. In response to this growing concern, a fresh crop of non-irritating, fragrance-, chemical- and soap-free formulations, with ingredients that evoke a calming effect like chamomile and aloe, have sprouted up over the last few years. These 'cosmeceuticals-lite' help restore and normalize self-inflicted reactive, red and irritated skin. Neutrogena was forced to add a 'sensitive skin' formula to their popular Healthy Skin AHA line to satisfy customer concerns. You would be hard pressed to find any cosmetics company today that has not yet introduced a product range specifically for 'sensitive, reactive or delicate' skin types. These Zen-like soothing formulas usually come bundled in pastel-coloured packaging with names like balm, pure and mist.

A common lament among dermatologists is that women often complain about having 'sensitive skin' which is hard to pinpoint. My first instruction for active skincare was in the mid-1980s. AHA technology was at its peak and plastic surgeons were beginning to dispense cosmeceuticals in their offices. I had memorized as much of the science as I needed to translate how glycolics worked and what they did, and learned with utmost precision how to determine whether a cream or a lotion was best and what strength to start the patient on. Just as I thought I had mastered the art of glycolic acid dispensing, the company's representative brought over a new product for me to test – a gel. I found myself in the unwelcome predicament of having to slip this new gel into the great cream v. lotion debate. Attempting to guide an already mystified group of women through the life-and-death decisions of choosing between a cream, lotion or gel should surely have earned me lifetime sainthood status. The basic regime was designed to begin at a level of 8% AHA and, once the skin was tolerating it well, we were instructed to bump patients up to 15%. When a few patients complained about redness and irritation, I was determined to work out what the culprit was. My careful probe into the situation revealed that these AHA fanatics were using the 15% on top of the 8% because they thought it would yield 23% acid that would work on their wrinkles faster.

If you use a wrinkle cream infrequently and end up with a fleeting redness, you might be tempted to classify your skin as 'sensitive' when it might not be at all. However, using 8% glycolic acid on top of 15% would make anyone's skin react unfavourably. Similarly, any acid after shaving is generally not a good idea. Truly sensitive skin is hyperactive or easily reactive, and can be sensitive to certain ingredients, especially fragrance and dyes. Skin can also react to climactic changes such as cold, wind or very hot weather, and also to over-hot showers. Although 'natural' sounds good for skin prone to reaction from the simplest formulas, even some botanicals that are supposedly naturally benign can be the cause of a reaction in true sensitive skin types.

Skin responds to the way it is treated, and redness, stinging and itching may be your skin's way of crying out for relief. Ms Tina Alster, Director of the Washington Institute of Dermatologic Laser Surgery, says, 'If you are too aggressive with your skincare regimen, you may aggravate reactive skin. Choosing a product that is inappropriate for your skin type or over-exfoliating can lead to inflammation or acne.' You probably wouldn't contemplate scrubbing your Le Creuset collection of cookware with a steel wool pad, so why would you rub grainy scrubs that feel like gravel into delicate facial skin? Although even sensitive skin needs exfoliation to keep its healthy glow, once or twice a week may be all it can comfortably tolerate. Fruit and botanical enzymes can be a good alternative to AHAs as an exfoliant for more reactive skin types. I once made the error of using Dior's Gentle Rose Exfoliant, one of the kindest light baby-pink facial gels with teeny particles, the morning after applying a hefty smear of Retin-A 0.05% cream all over my face. When I emerged from the shower my face was red and raw, and it took a few days of topical cortisone cream to calm down my self-inflicted scarlet cheeks. Another lesson in skincare learned.

Olivia Chantecaille
20-something, Creative Director, Chantecaille Cosmetics

- **What are your secrets of caring for your skin?**
  Daily spritzes of rosewater, regular applications of moisturizer, especially when flying, Shiatsu massage to decrease stress and not worrying that chocolate will give me pimples – because that's a myth.
- **How do you feel about the ageing process?**
  I live with my face and accept any changes, but if I can do anything to prevent ageing and feel good about how I look then I will.
  We are responsible for our bodies and nothing is forever.

- **Would you ever consider doing something for wrinkles?**
  I would do something against wrinkles if it were safe, painless and looked natural.

when in doubt, moisturize it!

If you consider which beauty product spends the most time on your skin, it would have to be your night cream. It should come as no surprise to anyone who has been shopping for skincare lately that night cream is also the most expensive single item in most product lines. One explanation is that the quality of the formulation has its effect dependent on how long it stays on the skin, and this, ultimately, determines how effective it is in rejuvenating the skin. There is something to be said for fine ingredients. Put them in a creamy base, add a little sensuous fragrance and a gorgeous jar with a jewelled top, and you can't beat it. According to Newby Hands, Health and Beauty Director of *Harper's & Queen*, 'Women using top skincare brands can see the difference. The implication that women are so stupid and vain that we will use something for years on end even though it has no effect, just because we've heard Sharon Stone buys it, is pure rubbish.' Although price alone is not a guarantee of superiority, it is equally unfair to jump to the conclusion that because it is expensive, it's a waste of money.

Night moisturizers are usually creams or lotions with a mixture of oil, water and various emulsifiers. They tend to be on the heavy side to protect the skin from the drying effects of night air, steam heat, central heating and air conditioning. Sometimes the difference between night and day formulas can be likened to consommé v. my granny's garden vegetable soup. Purists like me would never dream of using a body lotion on the face or a face cream around the eyelids, even though intellectually we know very well that it is not an act of cosmetic treason. The reverse, however, is quite acceptable. In my bedside table, too thick, greasy and perfumed face creams have been known to be relegated to hand creams after just one use. The most offensive versions are banished to the realm of moisturizers for the legs, elbows and feet. What you put on your face and around your eyes deserves special attention.

There is a simple rationale to this philosophy. Different kinds of skin have different weights and textures. Eyelid skin is the thinnest on the body. Facial skin is thicker, and body skin is thicker still. Different parts of the face or body have varying thickness and qualities, too. Most body cream formulas would be too heavy on the face, and face products can sometimes be too heavy around the eye area. The result may be that a too-rich face cream can leave the eyes looking puffy, which is somewhat self-defeating. Some face creams might be suitable for use around the eyes as well, but you can't be sure until you try it for yourself. Generally, it would be better to use a product specifically developed for delicate skin around the eyes, but to use it sparingly.

Many bedtime versions of moisturizers contain the word 'AGE' in the name or on the label, as night cream is rarely a staple of women under 30. Younger skins can get by without specific moisturizers for day and night. Night moisturizer varieties are specifically designed to appeal to the dehydrated faces of 'women of a certain age', or 'maturing women', as we are known in the advertising world.

Ultra-pricey luxury moisturizing creams de la crème have been cropping up with price tags of £100–200 per ounce and upwards. One of the most famous of these high-ticket creams is Crème de la Mer, developed by astrophysicist Max Huber with the exclusive magic bullet Deconstructed Waters. La Mer has a long list of devotees including Jennifer Lopez and Courtney Cox if that matters to anyone. A few other of the très haute moisturizers to add to your wish list are Sisleÿa Global Anti-Ageing (£150), Kanebo Sensai Ex-La Crème (£330) and Clé de Peau by Shiseido from the land of the rising sun. At £350 for Clé de Peau, you would expect them to send a beauty therapist named Yuko to your door every night to rub it in. La Prairie is right up there with their luxurious Age Management Stimulus, which is a retinol topping the charts at £120 and is so active that a Regular and Delicate formula is necessary. The same micro-sponge technology can be found in pharmaceutical-grade retinols, but that creamy lemon-yellow base and glistening silver pump container are clear marks of distinction.

Don't despair if £100 a jar will make a serious dent in your food budget. If it's moderately priced rich cream you seek, you will still have loads to choose from at the Clarins, Clinique and Lancôme counters, to name a few. Fortunately for us, the demand in the marketplace has caused technology to filter down to products you can find at your local chemist or supermarket, which offer age-defying, de-ageing and anti-ageing wunderkinds from Olay, L'Oreal, Nivea, Neutrogena and No. 7 – all bargains at about the price of a sandwich. I keep a Tiffany-blue jar of L'Oreal's Turning Point cream on my bedside table when I'm feeling particularly poor as a reminder that good things do come with smaller price tags so I don't feel deprived. Next time there's an unexpected ring at your door, if it's an Avon lady invite her in. Avon also has some of the best high tech creams around for about £12.

Women today not only have hopes for creams to be true miracles, we have GREAT EXPECTATIONS. We firmly expect formulas touted for their anti-ageing properties to live up to their promises, to work safely and gently and, above all, faster than the speed of light. We take a proactive stance in our quest for high performance skincare, especially if there is some kind of healthcare benefit that adds to its overall value. There is a segment of the female population that can be persuaded to fork over the gross national product of a small republic to pamper their skin, and the sky's the limit. However, the cachet and prestige alone of these creams is not enough to convince women to convert unless they really do something wonderful to the skin that gets noticed. We modern women buy our skincare now like we fill our closets; across lines of distribution, brands, seasons and price tags. While we may remain more loyal to our skincare brands than our lipsticks or eye shadows, if something better comes along, we're keen to try it. The quest for beauty in a bottle once separated women around the world by the barriers of price, geography and cultural differences. The Internet is becoming beauty's great equalizer, making beauty tools available to every woman with a debit card, no matter what corner of the globe she is in. Pricey beauty creams have been with us since the days of Cleopatra and they aren't going anywhere but up.

Creams de la crème

Some of my favourite de-ageing moisturizers and keratolytics (cell turnover promoters) that get high marks are:

DEAR BUT WORTH IT (£50 and up)

Morning
La Prairie Age Management Retexturizing Booster
Osmotics Kinetin Cellular Renewal System
Cellex-C Skin Serum
Sisley Hydra-Flash Formule Intensive

Evening
Christian Dior Capture Rides Multi Action Wrinkle Cream
Crème de la Mer Moisturizing Cream
Darphin Arovita C
Estée Lauder Advanced Night Repair

AFFORDABLE (From £20 to £50)

Morning
Estée Lauder Idealist
Lancôme Bienfait Total Fluide
Chanel Precision Age Delay Rejuvenation Serum
Clinique Stop Signs Anti-Ageing Serum

Evening
Juvena Q10 Triple Active Cream Night
Clarins Extra Firming Night Cream
Jan Marini Age Intervention Face
Helena Rubinstein Night Sculptor Line Lifting Cream

CHEAP & CHEERFUL (Under £20)

Morning
L'Oreal Plenitude Line Eraser SPF15
RoC Chronoblock Active Prevention SPF15
Neutrogena Healthy Skin Anti-Wrinkle Cream SPF15
Neostrata AHA Face Cream SPF15

Evening
Vichy Reti-C Concentre Nuit
Olay Total Effects Intensive Overnight Treatment
Avon Retroactive Age Reversal Cream
Helena Rubinstein Glycolic Exfoliating Lotion

so many jars, so little time
– a roll of the dice

With such a huge selection of possibilities on the market in every price range and method of distribution, the task of choosing the 'ideal' solution for your skin's needs can be daunting. The most commonly asked question about skincare in the age of beauty product overload is the ubiquitous, 'There are so many products on the market, how do you know what to choose?'

There is no definitive short answer to the question of what to use, and there are usually countless scenarios that would produce identical results. Every woman you ask will have her own personal recommendations – and women are usually flattered to be asked for their input. Ultimately, the process boils down to trial and error.

A beauty junkie's best friends are undoubtedly companies that give good samples. Although a foil sachet or a tiny bottle is never enough to be sure you're going to fall in love with the product, it is definitely enough to rule it out. If sampling is not an option, go directly to testers. At the very least it helps to test a product at the counter before you invest a small fortune in a skincare system or even just one jar of miracle cream. Ask to smell it, touch it and feel it on your skin. This is where some of the magic of buying skincare is lost on the Internet. The purely sensual pleasures of feeling and inhaling, the instant rush you get from bringing home a new beauty find and the anticipation of experiencing what it can deliver, remains somewhat lacking as retail therapy.

Unless you're a hardened beauty junkie (like me) with a medicine chest that runneth over, you probably need to get professional help. Seek the advice of a cosmetic dermatologist or an experienced and knowledgeable beauty therapist who can point you in the right direction. True skin authorities can see in a moment whether you need cosmeceuticals/medications and/or some other type of intervention to improve the condition of your skin – with or without mechanical assistance.

A Wood's lamp, skin scope or UV camera are common instruments of torture used to determine the levels of photo-damage, moisture or oil content in the skin. A thorough skin analysis by a professional can be a humbling experience, I'm afraid. You will never look at your skin with the same set of criteria again. I have always prided myself on basically good skin with little or no sun damage, based largely on the fact that I have spent the better part of my professional career behind doors (behind a desk would be more accurate). Then I had my photo taken with a UV camera at a dermatology conference and I became sadly enlightened. Every blip, mark, dot and dent was magnified into a life-size map of my personal sun history; that two-week holiday in Mustique, the sail in St Lucia with my ex-husband, the summers at Long Beach in my teens, the dutiful trip to Disneyworld with my daughter; there they all were, as large as life, if not bigger

Everyone in the beauty field has heard the refrain, 'I can't use it because I'm allergic.' It is usually said with the utmost authority and religious conviction. The truth is that unless a medical doctor specifically determines that you are allergic or overly sensitive to an ingredient, it may just be that you are using too much too soon. The woman who relates that she absolutely cannot use one ingredient or another can also be recalling a time when she slapped on globs of it without following the directions, or spent the day sunning herself after using it for the first time. If you are trying out a new skincare product, be careful not to use more than one new product on any body part on any given day. If you do have a reaction, the task of isolating the offending allergen will become practically impossible. High performance skincare, by virtue of its stated mission, has the potential to irritate the skin until such time as the skin gets conditioned to using it.

A sure sign that your skincare needs emergency assistance is when you begin to find that the products you have been using just aren't working any more. Your skin changes through the years and so do your skin's needs. Your skin can reach a plateau at a certain point and when it does, it's time for an adjustment. This can be as basic as adding a heavier barrier protection cream for a ski trek to Gstaad, or switching to an oil-free tinted moisturizer for a pending holiday in

Majorca. It can also indicate that your skin has become bored with the same old routine, and needs a jumpstart to shake it up a little. You can't expect to see revolutionary results from any skincare product overnight. By the same token, you can't expect to continue seeing results after years of the same boring skincare regime on ageing skin that is in a state of flux or decline. Although it is not practical to recommend an exact protocol for everyone, the Skincare Test below can clue you into surviving the skincare jungle.

Q&A: Skincare Test
If you answer YES to more than one question below, it's time to take your gold card for a spin!
1. Can you remember the last time anyone said how good your skin looks?
2. Does your skin often seem irritated, flaky or red in places?
3. Does your skin feel grimy or have a sticky residue or sheen?
4. Does your skin look dull or rough?
5. Do you get breakouts of spots that hang on for ages?
6. Do you find yourself piling on the foundation to cover up?
7. Have you used your current skin products in the exact same way for years?
8. Do you believe all skincare is the same so it doesn't matter what you use?

the mirror crack'd – repairing the image

In my 40th year I found myself evaluating facial rejuvenation procedures with a new set of criteria. My criteria became affected by my personal agenda: 'Would I have this done?' I often ask to observe surgery to keep up with new techniques in the operating theatre that I might have missed since I left the day-to-day administration of a cosmetic surgery suite in 1997. One of my visits was to watch Aesthetic Plastic Surgeon Alan Matarasso do a pair of facelifts at the renowned Manhattan Eye, Ear & Throat Hospital. MEETH, as it is known, has given birth to such world-class plastic surgeons as the now retired Thomas D. Rees and Michael Hogan, protégés of the late Sir

Archibald McIndoe, and a host of other giants still in the business of making women young and beautiful, including Sherrell Aston (Pamela Harriman's surgeon) and Daniel Baker.

At a benefit I had attended the evening before, my explanation for sneaking out before lemon sponge cake and coffee was that I had a date to observe surgery at the crack of dawn the next morning. I scarcely think anyone actually believed me, as they seemed to be eyeing me inquisitively over their Beef Wellingtons, wondering exactly what I was having done and why I had used such a lame excuse. My trusted assistant was not convinced and had earlier gathered up the nerve to ask me, 'You're not having surgery, are you?' Even to those unaware of my chosen profession, it appeared that I was a plausible candidate for facial cosmetic surgery. There was no chorus of the usual platitudes women hear from social acquaintances along the lines of, 'But you look great', 'You don't need anything done', and the ubiquitous, 'You don't have a line on your face.'

Protestations of this nature can usually be interpreted to mean that your dear friend and trusted confidante simply doesn't want you to look any better than she does. Looking good attracts other women to you. They are drawn by your sense of style, good taste and the confidence that comes with it. But there's a limit. If you look good, other women will ask you for advice on beauty issues. We will gladly tell each other about our experiences with a few office peels or playing at collagen shots, but we rarely come clean about the extent or details of precisely what, where and how much we've had done. For example, 'I've had a little BOTOX' may actually translate to 'a little BOTOX every three months for three years, and did I forget to mention the eye tuck and chin implant?' We are willing to share secrets about a sample sale or a great restaurant with far more candour than a 'hot' beauty treatment. When it comes to women and their cosmetic enhancements, the 'tell a little, keep a little' rule prevails.

Looking good throws the inimitable 'bitch' factor among women into high gear. It rears its ugly head when one among us is feeling insecure, threatened, vulnerable, jealous or just plain hissy. The relentless competition between girls over applause, friends, social invitations and male adoration begins at an early age. It's fine to look good, but not too good and definitely not too young. If you cross over the unspoken line of looking so good that you attract too much attention, especially from men, you are in grave danger of exile. Some women feel betrayed if you look better than they do. It is a form of rejection and you suddenly become the enemy. Looking great can be an immediate source of frost between females. If ever you feel the need to shake loose a few female friends, the surest ways are by dropping a dress size or two, dating a really fabulous fellow or having a facelift with all the trimmings. To hell with them! Who needs friends like that anyway?

Case history

Chatting over tea at The Connaught with Glenda, a 50-something publicist, and Pam, a cosmetics marketer in her middle 40s, I nearly gagged on my crumpet upon hearing Glenda exclaim that she was thinking of a lift. She is one of those rare, enviable women who personify perfectionism: the right bag with the right shoes with the great outfit that looks as if YSL fitted it to her body himself, and not a line, hair or mark out of place. No matter what I have on when we meet up, I always feel like an old hag in the shadow of her radiance. In the company of our mutual acquaintance, she talked about having had her eyes done some years ago but uttered not a single word about the lift I knew she had had done as well. Pam was surprised to hear that Glenda would even consider a lift, as it was obvious to all that she had nothing that needed putting back up or out on her face. After Pam departed to catch her train, neither Glenda nor I dared exchange even a glance on the subject of lifting again. I sensed that Glenda wondered whether I knew she'd had a lift, being a professional, but the admission has never passed her lips to this day.

3

dipping a
toe in the water

Youth is far from the only gauge by which good looks should be measured, and women no longer feel they have to be 25 years old to look great. If your goal is to stay well preserved, there is a whole category of treatments that stop just-short-of-the-scalpel. The ideal time to start thinking about dipping a well-pedicured big toe into these uncharted waters is before it becomes time to send up a flare. One measure is when people start saying 'You look a bit tired' or 'You look rather pale'. Personally, I loathe people who say that. It's really nothing more than a poorly disguised and polite way of saying 'Darling, you look like s—t.'

According to Mr Daniel C. Morello, Past President of the American Society for Aesthetic Plastic Surgery, '4.6 million surgical and non-surgical cosmetic procedures were performed in the US in 1999, which represents a 66% increase in the total number of procedures performed over the previous year. There was a 16% increase in surgical procedures and a 98% increase in non-surgical procedures including BOTOX, chemical peels, collagen and fat injections and laser resurfacing. We estimate the emphasis on less invasive techniques and combination procedures will continue well beyond the millennium.'

Wrinkle face map

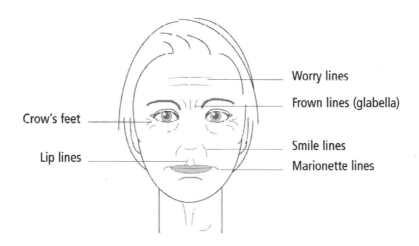

British attitudes about ageing
- 24% are worried about lines and wrinkles
- 47% are more concerned about wrinkles than retirement, loss of libido or children leaving home
- 53% of women only use a moisturizer
- 44% do not use any skin products
- 1 in 3 (30%) would undergo an anti-ageing treatment

(SOURCE: NOP survey of 1,100 women aged 25-65 years, May 2000)

Apart from the 'feel good' effects of pampering salon facials and aromatherapy massages that are delightful to indulge in but don't do much, the advanced, medically supervised treatments work deeper to produce visible results. Para-surgical procedures are 'look good' treatments because they actually do something, and bridge the gap between beauty salons and cosmetic surgery. If you are considering skin resurfacing, you need to decide how dramatic an effect you are really after. A light laser application, light chemical peel or just a home care programme may be enough. You can achieve outstanding results without subjecting yourself to pain and discomfort. The key is to distinguish between the dicey fads and the hype of pseudo 'quick-fixes' and the most effective and sensible treatments, in terms of the risks v. the benefits, value, results and time. The best candidates are anyone interested in improving the health and appearance of their skin.

What British women DON'T want from anti-ageing treatments

- Pain
- Scars
- Stitches
- Risks
- Blood
- Bruising
- Burns
- After-care
- Exorbitant Fees
- Down-time

When it comes to skin resurfacing, there is no substitute for experience. Whatever method or combination of methods you elect to have, it is critical to choose a technician who is experienced with that technique and knows all the nuances of it. There is a definite learning curve to knowing how to fine-tune the peeling solution or machine, control the depth of the resurfacing, and provide brilliant post-operative care. Often the level of risk rests in the hands of the technician rather than the nature of the procedure itself. Acids and lasers don't cause scarring; technicians who haven't properly learned the art of resurfacing do. Collagen remodelling is the proverbial pot of gold at the end of the rainbow of non-surgical anti-ageing procedures, and we will look at it in more detail in Chapter 4. It is the crowning glory, the ultimate achievement of a generation of research studies. Collagen remodelling is the formation of new collagen, which gives the skin a smoother, tighter texture and increases elasticity. The birthing of new collagen begins after the initial treatment and continues over time. In addition to recollagenation from lasers, peels and fillers, the other buzzword of the era is layering.

Layering is the process of using a combination of peeling solutions, lasers, BOTOX and/or fillers to get the maximum benefit from each. It's a matter of the total effect being greater than the sum of its parts. Layering has the potential to give a better overall result that lasts longer. For example, layering Zyplast collagen over Zyderm collagen, or Erbium laser over Carbon Dioxide laser. It also works well if you have several different areas to treat like fine wrinkles around the eyes, thinning lips, brown spots, and weathered skin all at the same time. Both of these concepts fall right in line with maintenance: the things you do before and after the lift or laser to get the most out of it and to make it last as long as possible until you're ready for the next lift or laser. The radiance of youthful skin is at a premium, but so is our time and how we choose to spend it.

Procedures for de-ageing your skin
Begin at the top in your 20s, work your way down the list through your 40s, have a lift, then start all over again.
1. Active skincare with OTC creams.
2. Superficial peels
3. Micro-dermabrasion
4. Medium peels
5. Skin rejuvenation laser treatment
6. Collagen Instant Therapy
7. BOTOX injections
8. Hyaluronic acid fillers
9. Fat transplantation
10. Some of the above again
11. All of the above again

The author's experience

As a matter of information, in case anyone is remotely curious, my face (b. 1959) is the very embodiment of anti-ageing layering. Note in the chart below my subtle graduation up the curve of beauty bits and shots as the years progress.

Year	Age	Beauty treatments
1994	35	Glycolic peels
1995	36	Began on Retinova cream
1996	37	Peel for lower eyelids
1997	38	Collagen to plump up lips
1998	39	Collagen to lips and nasal labial folds, BOTOX to the line between the eyebrows (known as the glabellar crease in the biz)
1999	40	Micro-dermabrasion, Collagen to the corners of the mouth and the crease lines starting at the sides of the nose and ending around the mouth (nasal labial folds)
		BOTOX to glabellar crease, Dermalogen (human tissue matrix, see Chapter 4) to nasal labial folds
2000	41	Micro-dermabrasion, hyaluronic acid to lips, nasal labial folds, fat transfer

wrinkle buster machines

If you're keen to have your lines and rough skin patches blasted mechanically, 'derma-peeling', 'micro-abrasion' or 'micro-derma-brasion' is making a big name for itself in the beauty world. In less than four years, micro-dermabrasion has skyrocketed to first place in the realm of skin rejuvenation techniques. It has become the opiate of beauty junkies everywhere and its overnight success can be credited to the low cost of the equipment and the unmistakable 'wow' factor it gives the face after just one treatment.

This is a non-surgical, non-chemical, non-invasive method of skin resurfacing. The newest microdermabraders are versatile, compact table-top units. They have a delicate tubular hand piece through which air is circulated to produce a stream of fine aluminum oxide micro particles that, along with suction, 'sand' the surface of the skin. This gentle skin blasting sloughs away the top dead skin layers and the results are equivalent to superficial glycolic peels.

The benefits of micro-dermabrasion are that it is safe for all skin types, there are few or no side effects, they are quick treatments that provide instant results and it is an affordable technology. Other benefits include not having to take any time off before or after the treatments. It is also an excellent pre-laser alternative and a good maintenance treatment for post-laser and peel treatments. Micro dermabrasion can improve acne, acne scars, superficial lines, superficial hyperpigmentation and scar tissue on the face, neck, back, hands and chest.

Dermabrasion (not to be confused with micro-dermabrasion) is performed with a patterned wheel attached to a hand-held rotary sander, resembling something you might find at a DIY shop. It has the potential to go much deeper into the skin and produce more significant changes in the skin texture – but it also leaves you looking a bit like you were turned upside down and scraped along the pavement. Lasers have largely replaced traditional dermabrasion, although it still works well for lines around the mouth and acne scars.

As with all superficial peels, a series of 6–8 micro-dermabrasion treatments is recommended at 2–4 week intervals. The number of treatments varies depending on your skin condition and the level of your commitment. Women like the results they get with these treatments and keep coming back for more, even after they have completed an initial series. The first time I had micro-dermabrasion I couldn't understand what all the excitement was. By the third or fourth, the unequivocal 'afterglow' effect hit home.

The micro-dermabrasion treatment should begin with a cleansing and degreasing of the skin. The approach is progressive, beginning on a mild setting using smaller size particles and eventually working up to higher levels and increasingly larger particles as your face becomes accustomed to it. The hand piece is applied to the skin, beginning at the centre of the forehead, moving out to the temples, following to the bridge of the nose, moving gently out along the cheeks, and finishing with the chin and around the mouth. It is generally begun with a horizontal pass, over which a vertical pass is directed, and ends with a circular pass to feather out edges and avoid visible grid marks or an area getting missed. It can feel oddly reminiscent of steel wool or fine sandpaper scratching off your dead skin cells. The more power used, and the more 'passes' or times the technician goes over a single area, the more abrasive it feels. Don't be surprised to feel a residue of crystals or particles sticking to your skin's surface and bits in your hair. A good brushing off and a spray of mineral water to refresh the skin after the treatments are advised. There may be a slight rosiness that most women rather like, but this is truly a 'lunchtime' procedure and you can apply makeup straight away.

Clinicians seem to be less impressed with the variable degree of improvement they see from micro-dermabrasion when compared with traditional peeling methods, but there is an immediate benefit after a single 30-minute peel. Savvy beauty junkies have discovered that if they schedule a treatment on a Friday afternoon, they can light up a room for a Saturday night out. With the exception of aggressive combination treatments that reach beneath the skin surface, and which should be relegated to doctors only, micro-dermabrasion is considered basically safe in the hands of a nurse, medical technician or beauty therapist. According to Rikki Allen, a nurse and aesthetic consultant from Sydney, 'Peeling and micro-dermabrasion treatments have been drifting into the domain of the medical aesthetician who has special training in skin physiology.'

The beauty of micro-dermabrasion is that it is a good multi-purpose skin resurfacing method that can stand alone or in combination with traditional glycolic peels to expedite results. Topical antioxidant serums or chemical exfoliants will also be able to penetrate the skin better once the upper layer of epidermis is sloughed off. As micro-dermabrasion technology gains credibility within the medical community, more clinical studies to measure the benefits on stretchmarks and on stimulating new cell growth will be done. Since the cost of the equipment is a pittance compared with other mechanical devices, we can expect a quick turnover of models featuring new bells and whistles at a rapid rate.

acid peels

The word 'peel' has been watered down to a catch-all term used to cover a wide range of treatments starting at the level of a mild glycolic wash from the chemist and ending with full-face Carbon Dioxide laser resurfacing. Any acid can be made to penetrate the skin lightly or deeply. The basic principles of peeling are: the deeper the peel, the better the result and the worse you look, the longer it takes to heal. The other critical variable is, of course, the person who is doing the peeling. Despite what you've been told, no peels are entirely idiot-proof.

You need to know what acid or acids are being applied to your face, even if you can't pronounce or spell their proper chemical names. You also need to have some understanding of the various factors that affect the peel result, such as the depth and concentration of the peel, how it is neutralized and the length of time it is on the skin. You may have had a 'peel' at a local beauty salon once or twice, but can't remember what or when, recall if you were red at all afterwards or whether you flaked, and couldn't necessarily pass a polygraph if pressed. On the other hand, some women will recoil in horror at the telling of the burning, itching and swelling from their last peel experience. Most Britons will simply say, 'It stung a little, but it didn't do very much.' One woman's 'sting' is another woman's 'burn'. The truth usually lies somewhere in between.

Chemical peels are flexible and can be adapted to various levels, depending on your needs. Apart from a basic skin classification (light to dark and tendency to burn or tan), the other factors in deciding what kind of peel to have (superficial peels v. deeper versions) are lifestyle-related. The distinction between a 'peel', 'facial peel' and 'laser peel' has been virtually erased. If you believe everything you read, it would seem that bottles of peeling solutions everywhere are being poured down the drain in record numbers in favour of micro-dermabraders and compact laser-like devices that have totally replaced traditional peeling techniques. Chemical peeling is here to stay, but like other skin resurfacing techniques, it goes through phases and changes with the times.

What to tell your doctor before you have an acid peel

- Your medical and surgical history, including: previous cosmetic facial surgery and resurfacing procedures (peels, dermabrasion, phenol, laser, etc), pregnancy.
- Your medication history, including whether you are taking antibiotics, anti-coagulants, have any drug allergies or adverse reactions to Roaccutane, Retin-A, Retinova, or if you are taking any herbal treatments or vitamin and mineral supplements.
- Your skin history, including scarring, radiotherapy treatments, chemotherapy, melasma during pregnancy, perimenopausal skin changes, acne, rosacea, psoriasis, eczema, herpes simplex, cold sores, cysts, incidence of skin cancers.
- Your lifestyle, including diet (vegetarians can have a higher risk of scarring), sun exposure, tanning bed use, smoking, nicotine substitutes, alcohol, sports and recreational pursuits (tennis, boating, gardening, etc) and your travel schedule.
- Your ethnic background (whether you are European, Mediterranean, Asian, Indian, African, Caribbean, etc) to rule out any history of or predisposition to post-inflammatory hyperpigmentation.
- Your skincare regime, including cosmetics and cosmeceuticals, your tolerance to active ingredients, your sun protection use, etc.

Your skincare expert should take an in-depth history and evaluation before he or she touches your face. As the 'peel-ee', you should also be eager to provide one. At each subsequent peeling visit, you should also update your peel-er on any relevant issues and changes in lifestyle, routine or skin condition since your last treatment. Your peel history should be well documented so that there is a record indicating pertinent details, including strength of solution, time left on the skin, hot spots that are more sensitive and any bad reactions. It is wise to find one skin clinic and stay with them so that your peel history can be monitored and progressively bumped up as your tolerance increases. If you flit from one clinic to another in search of the flavour of the month, you will have to repeat the process with each treatment.

Based on a comprehensive analysis of your skin, your doctor can help you clearly define what your goals are and present a variety of possible options based on what you want to get out of the peel, your tolerance for down-time and discomfort, and your budget. If you can't explain or identify what you want to improve or correct, it makes the job of selecting the appropriate peel that much more difficult and risky. According to Mr Andrew Clive Markey, FRCP, Consultant Dermatologist at The Lister Hospital, 'A wide range of skin conditions can benefit from chemical skin peeling. The critical steps are to determine the skin type, the nature of the condition requiring treatment and its depth in the skin (whether in the epidermis or the dermis), and tailor the strength and type of peeling agent used to reach the depth required.' For this reason, anything stronger than the most superficial glycolic peeling should be relegated to a medical setting.

Ideally you should be willing to accept the concept of a peel as a gradual programme instead of a one-time office treatment. If you plan to go back to sunning or tanning again, save your pennies and don't bother to have a peel at all. The details of the programme should be specified at the outset: how many treatments you will need (4–6 or more), at what intervals (2–3 weeks approximately), and what if any pre-conditioning and maintenance regime, including sun protection, is recommended. A typical superficial skin peel takes less than half an hour in total and the solution may be on your skin for only 1–12 minutes.

Peel spectrum

Peels range from the light to the deep and your choice will depend on many or all of the factors outlined above. Here's the lowdown on peels:

SUPERFICIAL PEELS

A light peel that must be done in a series to see results.
- Alpha hydroxy acids (glycolic , lactic, fruit acids) are considered the mildest of peel formulas.
- Beta hydroxy acid (salicylic) is a good peel for oily skin and spots.
- Jessner's Solution (resorcinol, salicylic acid, lactic acid, ethanol) can be used alone or in combination with AHA peels.

MEDIUM PEELS

These peels go slightly deeper and may be repeated.
- Trichloracetic acid (TCA). This type of peel is generally more effective than AHA peels on damage that rests in the deeper layers of the skin.

DEEP PEELS

These are usually a one-off event.
- Phenol or croton oil. These are aggressive peeling agents that have the potential to produce a more lasting effect.

For severely wrinkled or damaged skin, you will get a greater effect if you are willing to consider the trade-off of a slight disruption in your social diary. Most of us want the greater effect, but the notion of anything more than an overnight recovery is too long. Deeper peels with more concentrated solutions of AHA or Trichloracetic Acid (TCA) may take 5–10 days to heal, but the results will be more dramatic. Almost any skin type, even black, is a candidate for some form of chemical peeling, but the darker your skin, the fewer safe peeling options you have. The deeper the peel, the greater risk of having a bleaching or whitening effect (hypopigmentation), a line of demarcation and temporary as well as permanent scarring.

Beyond the physical examination lie the more subtle psychosocial aspects of the peel-er to peel-ee relationship. The underlying philosophy of entering into a peel programme is teamwork – the dermatologist, cosmetic surgeon and/or beauty therapist does his or her part, and you have to take responsibility for home care and maintenance. Home care includes sun avoidance and following the directions you were given on how to use post-peel products. Maintenance means sticking with it and having consistent peels, rather than one every now and then.

Après peel

Universal no-no's:

- Scratching peeled skin.
- Picking your face or pulling off scabs or crusts.
- Using abrasive skincare products too soon.
- Going into direct sunlight without a total sunblock and a hat and sunglasses (UVA/UVB/SPF30).

the laser conspiracy – rays, waves
and beams of light

The typical life cycle of technological advancements in cosmetic surgery is not unlike any other industry. Upon entering the market, gadgets and methods go through a period of review during which they are constantly refined. The language of the claims at this stage settles into moderation: 'permanent' becomes 'temporary'; '9–12 months' becomes '3–6'; and 'eliminates' becomes 'reduces'. Upon reaching maturity, a series of renewals, improvements and repositioning occurs to justify the hefty lease payments doctors will be making long after the technology is defunct. Cheaper models inevitably arrive on the market and occasionally the entire process is cut short when some unfortunate victim gets a bad scar and goes public, or the company goes under. In the end, the new technologies become the dinosaurs of tomorrow and the cycle begins again. Once 'cutting-edge-state-of-the-art' equipment eventually winds up for sale in the back of medical journals or on ebay.com. Products frequently come to market before doctors have had the opportunity to properly evaluate the risk v. reward ratio. Never was this truer than in the case of laser technology.

Lasers are destined to proliferate, and newer models are more compact, lighter, cheaper, easier to use, and capable of multi-tasking. As surgeons get more comfortable with combining resurfacing lasers along with surgery, more extensive lasering of faces and neck will become the norm. As technology gets better and better, lasers will be able to do everything from stimulating hair growth to curing acne to targeting fat cells with pinpoint accuracy.

Short of being an astro-physicist (aka rocket scientist), a layperson cannot begin to understand the bells and whistles of laser technologies. Each laser or laser-like device differs in its physics, energy, the way it works, and what it works on, and each doctor using the laser has the capability to customize the settings, pattern, time and depth of treatment. Basically, the vital statistics to laser resurfacing are how deep the wavelength goes and how many times the laser surgeon goes over the same skin surface. The deeper he goes and the more passes the laser makes, the redder you get and the longer you stay scarlet. Your choice is whether to go for one big procedure or several baby procedures to zap your wrinkles.

Typical laser treatment areas

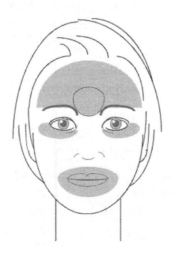

For laser resurfacing of the skin, there are 5 basic laser treatments. These are:
- Carbon Dioxide
- Erbium:YAG
- Coblation
- Non-Ablative Lasers
- Intense Pulsed Light

Carbon Dioxide

When lasers first hit the cosmetic scene in the 1990s, the manufacturers and used car salesmen who represented them led both doctors and consumers to believe that they were a no-brainer. Years later, there should be state-sponsored group therapy for some of the Carbon Dioxide laser's earliest victims who are now plagued by permanent scarring and skin lightening problems.

First on the market was the Ultrapulse produced by Coherent, which was quickly followed by a surge of other models. The investment in a laser is about £100,000, or as much as the price of a small cottage in Warwickshire. For that amount of money, you can expect a lot of wrinkles to be zapped, sometimes whether they need it or not.

The two most frequently used lasers for skin resurfacing are Carbon Dioxide (CO_2) and Erbium:YAG (see below). These lasers target the skin itself and the wavelengths are absorbed by water. Since most of our cells are predominantly water, these wavelengths are absorbed by the first cells they touch, i.e. the skin. When energy is delivered into the skin over a certain temperature, superficial tissues are vaporized and ablated or destroyed. Both lasers are used to resurface skin, but the CO_2 laser goes deeper and heats the tissues more than the Erbium:YAG. CO_2 is still considered the workhorse of lasers because of its ability to cause skin shrinkage (up to 30%), and its dramatic results on deeper wrinkles. Typically, after treatment you will be required to apply an occlusive ointment that water cannot penetrate for at least a week. The epidermis or superficial skin layer regenerates after that point, but the skin does not look altogether normal for a few weeks to a few months. The fairer your skin, the longer you will stay pink.

Erbium:YAG

Erbium:Yag (known as Er:YAG) technology has gained wide acceptance as the second cousin to Carbon Dioxide lasers, but without some of the side effects that most women are simply not willing to put up with. The Er:YAG is often used for sculpting deeper lines that remain after CO_2 resurfacing, as well as fine lines and wrinkles. New techniques combine Er:YAG with CO_2 to produce better results and speed up the long healing process that has turned many of us off the laser.

Few women have not had a friend or acquaintance that swears that she would never have a laser treatment again because of the oozing, scabbing, itching and redness. According to Professor Nicholas Lowe, 'What we've learned about resurfacing lasers over the last six years is that you should not be too aggressive. We are using the CO_2 and the Erbium:YAG superficially so that a woman can look good at about eight days, and the pinkness need not last more than a few weeks. If necessary, you can repeat it in a couple of years. You don't get the severe changes in colour and the whitening effects, but we can get good improvement.'

Coblation

Coblation uses bipolar radiofrequency (RF) technology instead of heat to remove wrinkled tissues with minimal thermal damage to the tissues around the wrinkles. It seals the blood vessels as it removes tissue and promotes skin tightening as a laser would but by a dramatically cooler process. Coblation is a less expensive resurfacing alternative that can sometimes offer faster healing, but the wild card is the long-term benefits on lines and wrinkles.

These systems are not regulated as strictly as lasers and are considerably less costly, so they could wind up in the hands of non-medical staff. Only have treatments under the supervision of a medical doctor who is trained in laser surgery – any laser can be dangerous in the wrong hands.

Non-Ablative Lasers

We have now entered the era of the day lasers, the kinder, gentler antidotes to facial wrinkles. The newcomer in the rapidly changing laser universe is 'cool ablation' or 'non-ablative' which emits a cooling spray to protect the epidermis (outer layer of the skin) before it heats the dermis (deeper layer), where new collagen is formed. The process of softening wrinkles continues over time as the rejuvenated skin fibres reach the skin surface. Non-exfoliating rejuvenating lasers like the Thermescent Laser Skin Treatment (CoolTouch) are gaining credibility as the waves of the future for younger women who want to prevent, postpone or maintain more invasive treatments. According to Professor Nicholas Lowe, treatments are done every 4–6 weeks over a 6-month period to maximize new collagen formation and should be performed beyond the actual area you want to improve; for example, lower eyes should ideally include the upper cheeks, to get a progressive tightening. Since non-ablative lasers have a very long wavelength, they are relatively safe for a variety of skin types. This technology is faster, recovery is shorter, there is less risk of pigment changes, and less or no pain. Although non-ablative lasers do not improve surface texture or remove brown spots, they are ideal for maintenance after more aggressive resurfacing, or as part of a total maintenance programme in combination with skincare and micro-dermabrasion. Another non-ablative system, N Lite Laser Collagen Replenishment, targets blood vessels in the dermis and safely removes wrinkles (from the peri-orbital area) without damaging the skin's surface. The patented technology, developed in Wales, is currently marketed in the EU and has received FDA approval in the United States. You're not going to see miracles from non-ablative lasers, but they work well as a basic anti-ageing treatment for superficial fine lines without any downtime.

Intense Pulsed Light

The new laser beams for all skin shades are cutting the red out. Another flash in our future is the Intense Pulsed Light (IPL), also called photorejuvenation, which is not a laser exactly, but a broad spectrum of pulsed light that can be used to improve age spots, enlarged pores, surface lines and spider veins on the face, hands, arms and neck. Marketed as the FotoFacial, this process is great for darker skin types. The treatments take half an hour, a series of

4–6 full-face applications are recommended, spaced 3 weeks apart, and you can wear makeup right away. IPLs work best for superficial flaws only, and are proving to be a good, gentle alternative for the laser-phobic.

Pre-laser skin rules
- Retinoeic acid (Retin-A, Retinova) may promote healing.
- For darker skin types, bleaching agents may be suggested.
- Take anti-viral medications to prevent cold sores.

Post-laser skin rules
- Use nothing except Vaseline or Aquaphor for the first 7 days.
- Use UVA/UVB sunblock – NO tanning or direct sun exposure.
- Wash with plain water, as directed.

laser regulation

The real problem in regulating who is allowed to use a laser in the UK, according to Professor Lowe, is that 'every separate health authority has its own interpretation of the rules. Some are very thorough and insist on laser physicists, doctors or nurses only, and safety officers will come round to check. With other health authorities, anything goes.' Keep in mind that where there is heat, there is a potential for a burn, and even supposedly fool-proof lasers can hurt you if they are used improperly. The other downside to having laser treatments with an inexperienced technician is the lack of adequate instructions and aftercare. There are some basic rules that apply when entering the laser-resurfacing realm. Lasered skin is much more prone to sensitivity and even the mildest of ingredients may cause your newly resurfaced face to react badly. Dermatitis and other irritations are common after resurfacing and can delay the healing process and make you miserable. 'When in doubt, leave it out' is a good premise to follow.

There is a recommended regime of preparing the skin to get the most benefit from the whole laser or peel experience. According to Rikki Allen, RN, 'The rationale behind pre-conditioning the skin is to remove the outer layer of damage to allow the use of less laser to get to the deeper damage so the skin will be less reactive following the laser treatment. Ideally, it should start a minimum of 4 weeks prior to the laser treatment. Skin preparation should consist of glycolic and retinoid creams morning and night and also sunblock, based on the level of sun damage. Post-laser, when the skin has healed, the collagen is in a state of flux for up to 4 weeks which can lead to milia, blackheads and acne.'

Case history

Julie Spenser, 53, read about a clinic close to her home that had the newest lunch-time laser peel. The doctor was a retired NHS consultant dermatologist engaged part time in the laser clinic. After being assured that she could get rid of her lines and wrinkles and that it was a simple procedure, Julie willingly signed up. After the procedure, the only instruction she received was to keep Vaseline on her face. Two days later she found herself oozing, encrusted with scabs and running a slight fever. Her husband insisted on taking her back to the doctor, but Julie felt too sick to do the 2-hour journey. She called to report what was happening, and her doctor stood steadfast in his belief that 'it was simply impossible to have that sort of reaction from a mild laser'. Several more days passed with no improvement, and her husband, fearing the worst, insisted that she call the doctor again. After a chorus of patronizing '…My dear's…' he told her to keep using Vaseline and she would be fine. Two months later, Julie went to see the doctor to complain about scars under the eyelids and around her mouth from the laser. He dismissed the ugly raised red marks as 'eczema', told her to put on a cream, and sent her home. Julie never had eczema before the laser peel, but she feared the wrath of questioning the doctor's authority.

The end result was that, contrary to what was told to her by the clinic doctor, she has permanent scarring that will require further treatment if it is to improve.

4

getting your feet wet

The quest for the 'ideal' wrinkle filler is a little like the search for the 'perfect' man. At some point you come to the realization that he doesn't exist and you settle for less. We are looking for a substance that embodies a host of traits that rarely co-exist in a given form at any point in time. Our dream filler should be safe, effective, predictable, easy to use, multi-purpose, long lasting and affordable. Finding that ideal combination of qualities is indeed a challenge for physicians, scientists and beauty junkies the world over. Women want maximum results with the minimum disruption and down-time, and to have their wrinkles filled during lunch. Luckily, fillers are the ideal combo treatment, and most can be mixed and matched as needed at one time or at a later date.

The original beauty shot was the mysterious medical-grade injectable liquid silicone popularized in Germany, Switzerland and Japan as early as the 1940s. The precursors to silicone included paraffin and flax oil that proved to be disastrous. My entrée into plastic surgery in the early 1980s made me privy firsthand to the Jekyll and Hyde personality of injectable liquid silicone (ILS). Along with power suits, oversized shoulder pads and Alexis Carrington jewellery, it was quite fashionable to have silicone shots for your lips, cheekbones, foreheads and skin folds.

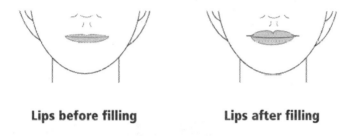

Lips before filling   **Lips after filling**

Legions of women took on the personae of drag queens in their pursuit of facial enhancements via the needle. Silicone was practically a black market substance that found its way into doctors' offices in the form of a clear, thick liquid. In those days, it was injected with a very large, threatening needle, without the benefit of a Valium or numbing cream. The modern micro droplet technique uses a more reasonable needle to place tiny drops strategically in the offending creases. Since liquid silicone was deemed 'illegal' in the US and France, there have been sightings around the world. (It is now approved in the US for very limited medical uses.) A favourite among vintage beauty junkies and some cosmetic surgeons, although many refuse to admit to it in public, silicone still has its share of advocates who swear that it is the only thing that lasts and that the droplets never migrate. It would be hard to ignore the hard knots and bumps that showed up months and years later. One thing appears to be certain; whether you like it or not, silicone is forever and it is nearly impossible to remove.

Today's beauty phenomenon is the sheer numbers of New York, LA and London elite who are beginning to look like they escaped from Madame Tussaud's with over-BOTOX-ed brows and exaggerated bee sting lips. As Mr Andrew Markey says, 'Permanence of correction is often seen as the Holy Grail for a filling agent, but just as fashions change, so does the desirability for lip fullness, brow position, cheekbone prominence and so forth. Permanent alteration can be less desirable than a temporary adjustable option.'

collagen nation

Survey a cross-section of women on what they want most in a wrinkle filler and you'll find that it's all about time and money. We want fillers that last because we don't want to be committed to multiple visits to a doctor's consulting rooms throughout the year. When given a choice, however, most of us generally prefer biological materials to synthetics, even though synthetics often last longer. Price is an issue because you could easily spend as much in a year on beauty shots as a facelift. Skin testing is a nuisance because the 'instant gratification' factor is delayed. Women want their wrinkles filled now, not a month from now, and we don't want to commit to returning for skin tests. Last but not least, heaven forbid the notion of anything more uncomfortable than a tiny 'pinch' or more than the mere shadow of a bruise!

According to Stephen Glass, Makeup and Enhancement guru at Fortnum & Mason, 'Many of my clients speak of having some sort of "treatment" in order to improve their appearance and a good number have had help via the knife. Generally speaking, English women are more conservative than their American counterparts and might start by having injections into lines and then the first "plastic" step.'

The ideal first step for a virgin beauty junkie who has just seen her first wrinkle is one of the' 'naturals', like collagen. In the wrinkle filler wars, collagen has proven to have staying power second only to autologous fat (your own fat, reinjected into your wrinkles). First introduced in 1977, injectable bovine collagen still holds the lead as the universal favourite among many physicians and patients. The concept of injecting substances to fill in facial wrinkles came into its own with the advent of Zyderm I. Later Zyderm II was added and finally Zyplast, which is the most substantial of them. Despite alternatives that have come, including porcine collagen derived from pigs, (which some might consider a waste of a good bacon rasher), none has withstood the test of time like collagen. Three decades later, it would be difficult to find a cosmetic surgeon in the world who has not had some experience with bovine collagen or who does not currently keep some in his office fridge. Part of the appeal of Collagen Instant Therapy, as it is now called, is the fact that it is versatile, predictable, safe and basically does what it is supposed to do. A series of two skin tests are required in the forearm and there is only a 3.0–3.5% reaction rate, which makes it safe for about 97% of women with wrinkles. If you haven't been treated or tested with bovine collagen within a year or so, a skin test is advisable to reduce any possibility of a reaction. Your body can change and develop a sensitivity to it, although it is rare.

Pre-filler preparation

Before you have any fillers, make note of the following:
- Inform your doctor of any history of bleeding and blood clots.
- Avoid aspirin for one week.
- Use a Vitamin K cream before and after to minimize bruising.
- Apply ice compresses immediately following treatment.
- Don't schedule your beauty shots around 'your time of the month'.
- NO fillers while pregnant or breast-feeding.
- Don't have fillers right before facial surgery – ask your surgeon first.

The biggest complaint among long-term collagen junkies is that it doesn't last. Exactly how much it doesn't last varies from line to line and face to face. Generally speaking, it doesn't last long and anywhere from 4 weeks to 4 months is not uncommon. The re-launch in

Europe of Collagen Instant Therapy conjures up two things; firstly that it does indeed fill your lines instantly, and secondly, that it is all too often gone in what seems like an instant. Collagen is the quintessential beauty maintenance product and it has to be topped up several times a year. To make it last longer, think layering. Combining Zyderm with Zyplast with other filler materials makes it last longer and fill better.

I have been dabbling with collagen since my mid-30s in the hands of a brilliant dermatologist, Dr Anita R. Cela. Up until fairly recently, I have been quite happy with the results, and although I'm not keen to have needles in my face, the 'ouch' factor has always been worth it. My personal theory about collagen is that it is lovely when you're in your 30s, but right around 40 it's a bit like the Dutch boy plugging up the dyke with his finger. As your lines morph into folds, it's time to put the troops on full standby.

The lowdown on collagen
- Possible side effects: Temporary bruising, swelling, allergic reaction.
- Average duration: 3–4 months.
- Beauty investment: £200–400 per area, per treatment.
- After treatment: Ice compresses.

If collagen from livestock doesn't strike your fancy, the runner up in the biological category is collagen from humans. This is where the science of tissue engineering is destined to play an evolving role in aesthetic medicine. The newer materials on the scene belong to a category of fillers known as 'allografts', tissues that are transplanted from one to another of the same species, i.e. 'apples to apples'. There are several human tissue grafts available in injectable forms (Dermalogen, Cymetra, Fascian) and implantable forms (AlloDerm, Dermaplant) that were first introduced in the mid-1990s, as well as Fascian, derived from human skin. The skin is donated to tissue banks for the express purpose of transplantation, and the materials are screened for Hepatitis, HIV and other nasty bugs. The tissues are then processed and packaged for medical use. The scientific theory behind allografts is that their biocompatible structure makes them a closer match to the tissue that has been lost, so it should last longer and may even stimulate the replacement of the graft materials with the body's own collagen. As the graft heals, it becomes part of your own tissue. These types of human injectables do eventually resorb and will have to be repeated or layered with another filler down the line. There is a world-wide trend afoot in off-the-shelf replacement materials towards biological or living tissues over synthetic components. If other people's tissue turns you off, grafts from your own personal fascia, skin and fat can also be used to plump up folds and creases.

In 1998, I was twice filmed having Dermalogen injected into my lips and nasal labial folds on camera for Munich Channel 7 and Brazilian TV Globo. Both producers were fascinated by the idea of human tissue being injected into wrinkles. My uncle emailed me to tell me his friend in Munich had caught a glimpse of me on television with a needle penetrating my lips. His friend hadn't seen me since I was at school and didn't believe I had any wrinkles to plump up. Although I consider myself to be a trooper in most vanity procedures, I thank God for the dental block used to numb me up before filming began.

Sunny Griffin
1960s supermodel and the original model for the Collagen Corp and now a youthful 60 and the CEO of Astara Conscious Skin Care

- **Are you still having collagen injections?**
  Not any more. I was 37 when Collagen did those ads and they used it all over my face. It hurt too much.
- **What are your top anti-ageing secrets?**
  I swear by self-tanners and don't go near the sun any more. I was a lifeguard in college, so I need to repair the damage. I eat raw fruits, veggies, nuts, living foods that have their life energy, and I still take ballet classes. I believe in natural organic botanicals, essential oils and major antioxidants like pycnogenol and Vitamin E. I try not to put any chemicals into my body or on my face.

- **What are the big innovations in beauty?**
  Today's skincare isn't 'Hope in a Bottle' any more, it has to be 'Results in a Bottle'. Women want products that do something for them. The other change is ethnic diversity among models.
- **Have you had any cosmetic surgery?**
  I had droopy eyelids very early, so I had to have them done for the camera at 34, 44 and 54, and I've had BOTOX twice. That's it for me.

hyaluronic acid gel fillers

Hyaluronic acid gels are quickly gaining recognition as the frontrunner in the next generation of fillers. Hyaluronic acid (HA) is a natural polysaccharide that exists in all living organisms, and specifically in the skin and connective tissues of the human body. Hyaluronic acid comes from the combs of roosters rich in HA, or can be produced biosynthetically through the fermentation of bacteria. The chemical structure of this substance is the same throughout nature, so it is very biocompatible and the body does not recognize it as 'foreign'. Although hyaluronic acid is not yet FDA-approved for wrinkles in the US, it carries the CE Marking of EU approval for a single-use product and has been distributed throughout Europe, Australia, Canada and elsewhere for several years.

There are many forms of hyaluronic acid fillers on the market and new models are continuing to be introduced all the time. The most common are Hylaform Viscoelastic Gel, distributed by McGhan Medical Corporation, and Restylane, a biodegradable injectable implant marketed by the Swedish biotech company Q-MED Esthetics. Hylaform is an injectable viscoelastic hylan gel treatment that is bio-engineered to simulate natural non-animal material. It is has a long shelf-life and does not require refrigeration. There is no skin testing for an adverse reaction required, so it offers the agreeable option of just a one-visit treatment. Depending on who you ask, it appears to last longer than bovine collagen, in some people as long as 6–8 months.

Hyaluronic tonic

- Possible side effects: Persistent swelling, tenderness, bruising, acne.
- Average duration: 3–6 months.
- Beauty investment: £200–400 per area, per treatment
- After treatment: Ice compresses

Restylane is the first stabilized Non-Animal Hyaluronic Acid (NASHA) that becomes fully integrated into the body. It is non-animal, so there is no chance of an allergic reaction. Q-Med obtained CE-mark approval in 1996 for Restylane and in 2000, they launched two new HA cocktails; Restylane Fine Lines for superficial lines around the eyes and lips, and Perlane, a thicker formula for deep facial contours and lip augmentation. These fillers are based on Q-Med's 'Tissue Tailored' concept; each is designed to be injected at a specific level in the skin to match the tissue structure at the level of injection.

None of the HA fillers contain a little thing called lidocaine, a numbing agent that you get in collagen, so it is not pain-free. The layering technique can also be used with HA to make it last longer. Treatment with hyaluronic acid should only be administered by physicians or registered nurses under medical supervision. Clinical trials are under way for Hylaform and Restylane in the US, and hope springs eternal that they will be approved soon so that plane-loads of American women won't have to turn in their frequent flyer miles to have it done.

Fillers are like coaches; a new one comes along every 30–40 minutes. There is a rapid unregulated approval of filling substances throughout Europe, according to Professor Lowe. 'All that is required is a limited amount of testing to show that their product has the equivalent immediate filling ability as an existing product, which makes for numerous fillers entering the market before they should be approved for use in patients.'

Another multi-purpose filler with a good safety record originated in Belgium is marketed under the name New-Fill®, made from microspheres of poly-L-lactic acid, the material found in cat gut sutures. It is totally bioabsorbable, which always makes me happy, and is designed to stimulate the body's own collagen for several months after the treatment. The good news is that the product is mixed for each patient, so anaesthetic can be added to the syringe.

Funky fillers from synthetic components and acrylics

- **Aquamid** Synthetic polyacrylamide gel
- **ArteColl** Microspheres of polymethylmethacrylate (PMMA), which is used in dentures and hip prostheses, suspended in bovine collagen. The collagen degrades in 3 months, and some of the PMMA beads may last after each treatment. Persistent swelling and lumps have been known to develop.
- **Dermadeep** Larger molecules of acrylic hydrogel
- **Dermalive** This filler from France is similar to ArteColl but has PMMA particles of different sizes and shapes suspended in a base of hyaluronic acid instead of bovine collagen.
- **Evolution** Porous polyvinyl acylamide microspheres in a gel

Mr Andrew Markey cautions, 'An ever-increasing number of skin filling agents is becoming available. However, it takes time to establish the true frequency of side effects and long-term safety of newly released compounds. The latest product is not always the best, and it is often many months before doctors can clarify the advantages and disadvantages of any new filler compared with existing products.' If tried and trusted fillers are what you want, stick with collagen, the hyaluronic acid fillers that have been around the longest, and fat, since you know where that comes from and there will be no foreign bodies floating around to cause you worry down the road.

fat recycling

What woman alive hasn't at one time or another fantasized about taking fat from her hips or bum and sticking it into her cleavage? If you are keen to plump up your wrinkles and folds with your own stuff, fat recycling may seem like a dream come true. Most women, with the possible exception of Calista Flockhart and Jemma Kidd, have enough body fat to fill 'er up on demand. There are several body areas that work well as fat donors, including the obvious places like the abdomen, buttocks, hips, outer thighs and knees. Sadly, to date, there is no method of loaning your excess fat to a deserving fat-less friend, although I wouldn't rule it out for the future.

The French are credited with starting the fat revolution in the first place. Although fat grafting has been used for over a century, it was nearly forgotten until the father of liposuction, the now retired Parisian plastic surgeon Yves-Gerard Illouz, gave fat its renaissance in the late 1970s. The techniques he and fellow fat pioneer Pierre Fournier developed for harvesting fat became widely adapted for transplanting it as well.

Fat grafting

- Possible side effects: Lumps or unevenness, bruising, swelling.
- Average duration: From 2 months to 12 months with some permanence after each treatment.
- Beauty investment: £300–£2,000 depending on extent of treatment.
- After treatment: Ice compresses, fingertip massage.

The driving force behind the flood of volume replacement techniques is the fact that you start losing fullness in your face after age 25. By replacing the lost volume with fat, an old, gaunt face can actually be made to look younger. Ageing robs us of our rounded cherubic cheeks and the fullness in our faces. Gravity causes the skin and muscles of the face to slump, the soft tissues to break down, and skin to lose elasticity and moisture content. Sliding and sinking set in, and sagging cannot be far behind. The trend in modern aesthetics is to preserve or replace facial fat to maintain the curves of a young face, instead of removing every last drop which can skeletonize you. Sharp lines and bony contours without the benefit of soft, healthy tissues can be very ageing on a woman in her 40s. If you have a plump face to start with, this may not be much of an issue for you.

The fat recycling process involves three distinct stages: harvesting the fat, storing the fat for future use and the actual injecting of it. Doctors rarely agree on what the perfect fat technique is, how long it can last, how many treatments are needed, to freeze it or not to freeze it and what to do about lumpiness. The variables include how the fat is extracted, what area is injected, how deeply it is injected, how much is used, the age of the patient, skin thickness, and who is doing the injecting. Getting two cosmetic surgeons to concur on the best recipe for fat transfer is as unlikely as Tory and Labour shaking hands on issues concerning the European Union.

Dr Patricia Wexler, Dermatologist to Donna Karan, Barbra Streisand, Ellen Barkin and supermodel Stephanie Seymour.

- **What are your secrets for smart ageing?**
  Start young, do little procedures frequently, and don't save it all up for later. You should enjoy your face while you're still young.
- **What are women looking for today?**
  I did a survey of my own patients and the average age that they become unhappy with their looks is 43, when they start complaining about the jawline and the neck, changes in forehead creases, nasal-labial folds and the angles of the mouth. Women today want 'wash and wear' procedures, and most people are candidates for combination treatments.
- **What advice do you give to women who want the latest quick fix?**
  Ask a lot of questions first. I never want to be the first or the last to try something – I like to be somewhere in the middle. You may look great for the first year or 2, but how you're going to look 5 years down the road as your face ages is what concerns me.

- **What are your favourite fillers?**
  Collagen is a great filler, hyaluronic acid gel is good for deeper corrections, and fat is the BIG filler that plumps up creases and folds.
- **Would you lift and tell?**
  I've been having BOTOX for 10 years on my furrows, and I had a full-face TCA peel in my 20s and one in my 30s. I love Hylaform and I did a CoolTouch laser treatment when I first started using it on my upper lip lines, which have always been my trouble spot.

Since the 1990s, a number of cosmetic surgeons world-wide have advocated a zealous use of autologous fat (your own fat) for every conceivable cosmetic purpose for the face, body, and hands. These 'fat Nazis' have created a virtual explosion of enlightenment over fat transplantation applications, but fat is not the universal answer for every flaw. It works on some and doesn't work on others, and the ones who need fat put back into their faces the most usually have the least of it to spare. When there are a number of ways of doing something, and they all come out about the same, it probably doesn't make that much difference.

Like all injectables, fat lasts better in static lines rather than in mobile areas like around the mouth, which is subject to the variables of animation, yawning, puckering and chewing. Fat is also not a one-shot deal and several treatments are needed for staying power. The further away from the mouth the fat is placed, the better it takes, and the efficiency increases with subsequent injections; that is, if 30% lasts after the first treatment, 50% may last after the second, and more after the third.

Fat grafting is performed under a local anaesthetic and can take from half an hour to several hours, depending on the extent of the procedure. There is an ongoing debate over the pros and cons of frozen fat v. fresh fat. Syringes of fat can be injected immediately or stored in zipping storage bags with your name, date and identification code at a temperature of about $-8\,^{\circ}C$. The syringes needed for your monthly or bi-monthly fix are defrosted at room temperature for a quarter of an hour before injecting.

Fat can work wonders to fill out deep folds around the mouth, hollow cheeks, eye sockets, deep scars and pointy chins. As Mr Andrew Markey says, 'Fat does not replace a facelift, it does something a facelift cannot do. If your skin is loose and hanging, fat alone is not the best choice. You may need a lift to tighten the skin.'

The future of liposuctioned fat tissue holds the promise that it may soon provide the raw material to manufacture new tissues. Results from numerous studies have led plastic surgeons to conclude that human fat tissue contains 'stem' cells that can potentially be turned into bone, muscle, cartilage, fat and other tissues. While the technology is not yet universally available, this research may have major implications for the treatment of 'tissue excess' states like corpulence, 'tissue loss' states like osteoporosis and ways to control tissue growth. It may also develop new techniques for breast augmentation using your own tissue instead of an implant. It seems only fair to me that all women should get a tax rebate for their environmentally conscious recycling efforts.

One of my favourite fat addicts, Heather Jones, received an announcement that her doctor was moving her practice miles away to another area. She immediately rang up the doctor's surgery to make sure they were taking all of her precious frozen fat with them on the move. Heather's rationalization for eating more than she probably should is, 'I have to keep eating to have enough fat for my lips.' Perhaps the best thing about fat is that most of us have an unlimited supply and it's free.

filler philosophies

There is more than one way to treat a line or a wrinkle. The beauty of fillers is that they can safely be combined with other treatments including BOTOX, chemical resurfacing with peeling solutions and laser technology, as well as rejuvenating surgery. Fillers also maintain the results of surgical intervention for the long term. Here's a summary of how often you might need to fill your lines:

Age and depth of lines	Treatments per year	Filler options (solo or layered)
30–40 (Superficial lines)	2–3	Collagen, Restylane Fine Lines
35–45 (Medium lines and creases)	3–4	Collagen, Restylane, Hylaform, Fat
45 + (Deep creases and folds)	3–6	Restylane, Perlane, Hylaform, Fat

FAQ's about injectable fillers from Fill-ees to Fill-ers:
- What is the source of the material (natural or synthetic)?
- How long has it been on the market?
- What kinds of clinical studies have been done?
- What are the possible side effects?
- Is skin testing required?
- Can I be allergic to it?
- What does a reaction look like and how long does it last?
- What can be done if I have a reaction to it?
- How long will the filler last?
- How many treatments will I need and how often?
- How much will each treatment cost?
- What are the risks?
- If it doesn't look right, what can be done to remove it?
- Can I still have other fillers later on?

the miracle of BOTOX

Botulinium Toxin Type A, or BOTOX, as it is affectionately called by those of us who live and breathe it, is not a filler like collagen or fat. It is actually a potent neurotoxin derived from bacteria that is used in minute amounts to soften wrinkles known as 'dynamic' (i.e. in motion) caused by the contraction of a facial muscle. The aesthetic benefits of BOTOX were discovered quite anecdotally by

BOTOX injection

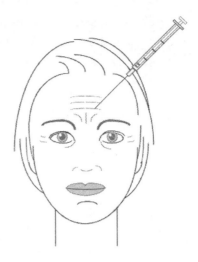

ophthalmologist Jean Carruthers and her dermatologist husband Alastair Carruthers in Vancouver in 1988. One of Dr Jean's patients suffered from blepharospasm, a spasming of the eyelid muscles, and begged her to treat the frown area between the eyes (glabellar area) with BOTOX, which she would not have normally treated since it was not spasming. The patient protested because her family always said that she looked so rested and untroubled after the BOTOX injections to that area. Of course, Dr Alastair had a lot of patients with glabellar frown lines that he had been treating unsuccessfully with alternative treatments. As the Carruthers say, 'The essentials were a chance remark, Jean's alertness to the remark and her skill with BOTOX, and Alastair's cosmetic practice.' That is how a generation of BOTOX junkies was born, and the rest is history.

BOTOX weakens the facial muscles that create wrinkles and frowns when they contract. The injections take just minutes and are done in the clinic with nothing more than a local cream anaesthetic. BOTOX comes in a glass vial containing 100 units and is diluted with sterile saline before use. It may take from 2 days up to 2 weeks to have a full effect, and a touch-up treatment may be needed later if the muscles are still active. A small number of unlucky women have muscles that are resistant to BOTOX and too many treatments with large amounts of BOTOX can cause you to produce antibodies to it, although it is rare.

BOTOX me

Top 3 BOTOX uses according to Alastair Carruthers, FRCPC:

1. Prevention of frown lines.
2. Treatment of crow's feet.
3. Horizontal forehead lines.

Dr Carruthers says, 'The average ageing individual tends to be slightly more concerned about crow's than frowns, and there seems to be an emphasis on crow's feet in sunnier climates and frown lines in less sunny climates. However there is a hard core of frowners for whom BOTOX is essential to their ability to express themselves accurately.'

A wee bit of BOTOX does a really powerful job, but it is never permanent and has to be repeated every 3–6 months. When it starts to wear off, muscle activity will gradually begin to reappear, so you won't wake up one morning to all of your pre-BOTOX wrinkles lunging at you in the bathroom mirror. The goal of BOTOX is a subtle softening, not necessarily the complete elimination of facial expression lines. Very small amounts of this precious solution are injected to paralyse the muscle. A cosmetic surgeon who is adept at injecting BOTOX strives to utilize the least amount of toxin needed to get the job done. Accurate dosages and precise positioning of toxin is critical to freeze the right muscles just enough. BOTOX is too precious to be wasted. In the early years, there were incidents of temporary drooping of one or both upper eyelids that scared many women away. The electromyographic technique was developed to guide doctors to exactly the right spot in the belly of the muscle to position the tip of the needle prior to injection. Although electromyography (EMG), a method by which the muscles are isolated so that the surgeon knows exactly where to put the BOTOX, is not required, some doctors consider it a useful learning tool, especially for beginners. Done correctly, drooping occurs in less than 1% of all BOTOX treatments.

The BOTOX solution
- Possible side effects: Temporary bruising, headache, drooping, unevenness.
- Average duration: 3–6 months.
- Beauty investment: £200–500 per area, per treatment.
- After treatment: Stay horizontal for 4 hours, flex your muscles, apply ice if desired.

'If my patients have a muscle that's even thinking about twitching, they want it frozen,' says San Francisco Dermatologic Surgeon Mr Seth Matarasso, 'but sometimes it's a matter of too much of a good thing. When it comes to BOTOX, "less is more" prevails.' If BOTOX is injected beyond the midpoint of the brow laterally towards the temples, brow 'ptosis' (drooping) can occur. This drooping is temporary, but it can present a real nuisance if you have a big date or event coming up before it subsides. If your whole forehead is treated with BOTOX to eradicate every last horizontal line or furrow, the position of the eyebrows may drop, and create a crowded eyelid area. If your brows are low to begin with, BOTOX can be used as a 'chemical browlift' to raise your arch ever so subtly. Too much BOTOX, popularized by the frozen faces of starlets at the Cannes Film Festival or the Academy Awards, can result in a very flat, vacant, expressionless look.

Over the age of 30, there aren't many women (or men) who wouldn't benefit from a little BOTOX shot to their frowns and furrows. BOTOX injected into the glabellar region paralyses the muscles that enable you to frown. By relaxing these muscles, many doctors believe that you can actually slow down your brow descent and prevent the deepening of a glabellar crease. The theory in vogue is to start your BOTOX before your creases are so deep that they need to be filled up with collagen or fat in addition to your BOTOX therapy.

There are two forms of botulinum toxin B on the market; BOTOX is marketed by Allergan Inc (Irvine, California) in the US and 61 other countries, and Dysport from Speywood Pharmaceuticals Ltd (Maidenhead, England). The US version is freeze-dried and the UK version is freshly made and more concentrated so it requires more dilution. Botulinum toxin B is marketed under the brand names NEUROBLOC in the US and MYOBLOC in the EC, both from Elan Pharmaceuticals. This form does not require dilution and is considered to be more potent. The more BOTOX you need, the more expensive your treatment will be as well. There is a definite learning curve with BOTOX injections, and the more a physician works with it, the more finesse he develops in determining precisely how much to use and where to put it.

BOTOX has been found to work for fine lip lines, drooping corners of the mouth, nasal labial folds and chin wrinkles, although in a more limited way. The future of BOTOX for the signs of facial ageing is unlimited. According to Dr Jean Carruthers, 'We are still learning how to use BOTOX on the mid and lower face. Increasingly, doses into the lower eyelid and lips are becoming popular. Treatment of the sad lines at the corner of the mouth will also be a useful adjunct to other treatments such as injectable fillers.'

The beauty of soft tissue augmentation is that it can safely be combined with other treatments, including BOTOX, chemical resurfacing with peeling solutions and laser technology, as well as rejuvenating surgery, to produce a more natural overall result. Fillers also maintain the results of surgical intervention for the long term, but no one of the available agents is applicable to all defects. New and improved fillers are going to be the way of the future.

Case history

Rosa Latham, 47, hated having hooded eyes. She went to see a top eye surgeon who suggested that the excess skin and fat of the upper lid could be removed to open up the eyelid area. She had surgery which turned out fine but a year later, she felt her lids getting droopy again. She assumed that more skin needed to be removed from her eyelids. What she didn't realize was that she was a victim of BOTOX overload. Helen had had BOTOX injected into the frown lines between her brows. The doctor treated the lines on her forehead too but it had been injected all across her forehead lines, causing her eyebrows to fall down. This defeated the original surgery that was supposed to open up her eyelid area.

5

two toes...

The missions of modern cosmetic surgery are two-fold; to achieve the most satisfying improvement with the least amount of surgery, and to minimize the conspicuous signs of surgical enhancement. 'Minimally invasive' surgery should never be confused with 'non-surgical'. Any time a surgeon makes an incision, it's real surgery. According to Mr Gavin Morrison, President of the Association of Plastic and Reconstructive Surgeons of Southern Africa, 'The trend towards less invasive surgery is driven mainly by patients who, understandably, desire less visible scars.' Many women simply cannot afford to devote the additional time required for more aggressive procedures. The alternative is accepting a less dramatic result from the lighter procedure that can always be repeated if needed down the line.

The advent of having a smaller surgical procedure done more frequently from the 30s onwards, instead of waiting until your neck and jowls are resting in your lap, is undoubtedly the wave of the future. According to Dr Donald Wood-Smith, 'The ideal patient for an extended minilift is between the ages of 40 and the mid50s, who has looked good up until recently, and is now beginning to get comments like "...You're looking tired". The end result replaces anatomic structures where they once resided and leads to comments like, "You must have wonderful genes" or "I've never seen you looking so well".' The results of modern techniques for modified and short scar facelifts can be compared with traditional procedures with their longer scars and healing times. In cosmetic surgery, it's all a matter of the trade-off.

According to Mr Alan Matarasso, 'The traditional facelift requires a continuous incision that starts 2–3 inches above the ear in the temple, then down in front of the ear for 2–3 inches around and into the crease behind the ear with an extension to the hair behind the ear, which adds up to about 8 inches in most people. The modified or short scar techniques cut the scar down to 3½ inches, or about fifty per cent.'

The more modern methods are most innovative in the length and positioning of the scars. Instead of making an incision into the hairline in two places, the newer methods stop before the incision gets into the hairline. 'The incisions that give patients the most problems are the one that lies in the crease behind the ear and the one in the hair. This procedure eliminates most of that,' says Mr Matarasso. For busy women with children, careers and better things to do, like most if not all of us, even a few days less of healing time can make a difference between being able to have a facelift in the narrow window of time you can set aside, or having to put it off for a year or two.

Modified or limited incision lifts have the advantage of a shorter recovery and can be applied to different scenarios (including men) and, most importantly, visible scarring and the incidence of changes to the hairline are greatly reduced. According to Dr Bryan Mendelson, 'Minimally invasive surgery changes the ideal time at which to commence surgery. Using modern techniques, the patient will have a better and more natural result by being operated upon at a younger age, when the deformity is becoming apparent but not fully developed. The end result is that the patient has a refreshed appearance, rather than waiting till they have an older appearance and the surgery makes them look younger again. There are obvious psychological benefits in avoiding the awareness of ageing changes of the face.'

Newby Hands, the 30-something Health and Beauty Director of *Harper's & Queen*, shares her thoughts on lifting, lasers and life after 30.

Fighting the ageing process can be confusing; apart from the surgical options, there is a constantly expanding market of high-tech skin treatments, both medical and surgical, new line-filling substances plus all those high-tech creams to rejuvenate the face. The best advice is to keep it simple and clear-cut, and always make sure you get the best advice and only work with the most experienced professionals. Also, don't fall for the gimmicks – remember if a doctor or surgeon is boasting that they are the only one to be doing a procedure there is probably a good reason why no one else is using it. So stick to what is tried and tested so you know it works and, more importantly, that it's safe.

shades, drapes and windows to the soul

The eyelids are the window shades for your eyes; they provide a frame through which the world views your most expressive feature. Their job is to protect the eyes from light and wash away dirt and irritants with every blink. Fat around the eyes cushions the eyeball and the muscles open and close the lids. Eyelid surgery should never compromise the functional elements of the eyelids for the sake of aesthetics. Your eyes are one of the first features people notice and, regrettably, they are also among the first to show signs of ageing.

If you had to pick the one area of the face that doesn't wear well, it would be the delicate and thin tissue around the eyelids. It is also subject to the most abuse, such as endless ordeals with waterproof mascara, liners in bottles, smudgy pencils and wands, smoke-filled rooms, popping in contact lenses, bawling and eye cream overkill.

The eyelids age in a couple of ways. Constant exposure to the sun without the protection of wraparound Gucci sunglasses will have a direct effect on the weakening of the elastic fibres that keep your eyelid skin taut. Droopy eyelids (ptotic in doc speak) or puffy lower eyelids often run in families. Protruding fatty tissue from your eye sockets that causes bags can be an inherited trait that shows up early in life, as well as the result of ageing. At first, bags or sagging may be most noticeable when you are particularly tired, and then the signs become visible all the time. Upper lids become heavier and fuller and crêpey skin may start to hang over the eyelashes. Some eyelid surgery falls within the realm of medical necessity, especially when excess skin overhangs part of the eye and interferes with your field of vision.

Dark circles and under-eye puffiness are two separate problems. According to the British Association of Dermatologists, 'Unlike the majority of "flawless" faces presented by the media, few of us have access to professional makeup artists or computerized image enhancement and many people worry about their skin tone or variations within it. There are normal variations in skin colour in all races. For example, the skin below and around the inner corner of the eye is often darker.' Dark circles can be a vascular problem caused by dilated blood vessels under the eyes. Some women are predisposed to bags, while others can look blue or black under the eyes from sinus congestion and allergies. As the skin is so thin under the eyes, any discolourations show through. Under-eye puffiness is caused by fluid and fat. Puffiness results when a fat pad that cushions the eye begins to pull away from the bone of the lower eye and sags. Gravity has its effects on the eye as well. Retaining water can cause puffiness, especially in the morning as water redistributes to the head while you sleep. Your affair with the salt shaker may contribute to under-eye puffiness as well.

For eyes that have it

Specially designed eye-care products are best to use on the eye area, but avoid heavily fragranced and super greasy creams.

- Don't drag, tug or stretch your saggy eyelid skin.
- Use only soft, pure cotton wool pads around the eyes.
- Always remove your eye makeup at bedtime.
- Don't apply eye cream to the upper eyelid.
- Use only small dots of moisturizer around the eyelid area.
- Never rub the cream into the skin, pat on lightly.

Eye creams for dryness and fine lines

- La Prairie Cellular Contour Eye Cream
- Helena Rubinstein Eye Sculptor Line Lifting Cream
- Shiseido Benefiance Revitalizing Eye Cream
- Elizabeth Arden Millennium Eye Renewal Cream
- Caudalie Grapeseed Eye Contour Cream
- L'Oreal Plenitude Line Eraser Eye
- Nivea Visage Coenzyme Q10 Wrinkle Control

Eye gels to help soothe and de-puff

- Lierac Dioptigel
- Molton Brown Eye Rescue
- Clarins Eye Contour Balm
- Cellex-C Eye Contour Gel
- Philosophy Dark Shadows
- Joey New York Lift Up Eye Gel
- Olay Revitalizing Eye Gel

Once or twice a week treatments

- Lancôme Primordiale Intense Crème and Eye Treatment
- Shu Uemura Skin Care Moisture Eye Zone Mask
- Samuel Par Eye Contour Concentrate
- Decleor Contour Mask for Eyes & Lips
- Erno Laszlo Firming Eye Gel Mask
- Dr Hauschka Eye Solace
- Biore Fine Line Gel Patches

The goals of eyelid rejuvenation techniques are to remove excess skin and fat, to re-establish the crease in the upper lids and to correct slack muscles of the lower eyes that pull the lid down. The lower eyelids have 3 pockets of fat under each eye. This type of fat won't respond to a low carb diet and pilates, but requires a headlong retreat to the cosmetic surgeon. The good, and sometimes bad, news is that fat pads around the eyelids tend not to grow back once they are removed. Eyelid skin is notoriously unforgiving and, as such, the overriding mission is to maintain the natural shape of the eye rather than to change it. If you weren't born with almond-shaped eyelids, it is probably because genetics wasn't in your favour. Asking to have the shape of your eyes changed is looking for trouble. According to Dev Basra, FRCS, 'It is critical not to distort the natural lines and gentle curves of the eyelids. Little sophisticated changes can bring about major improvements.'

Is it time yet?

Signs that you might need your eyes done:

- You can no longer locate the crease on your upper lid.
- You start investing heavily in progressively darker and larger sunglasses.
- No amount of thick black curling mascara makes your eyes look big any more.
- You can't remember the last time anyone told you that you have nice eyes.
- The puffiness under your eyes doesn't go away after the morning passes into midday.
- Cucumber slices and tea bags don't do the trick any more.
- You've cut your hair into a fringe to cover your eyes.
- You wear your reading glasses even when you're not reading.
- You get a headache trying to pick your eyelids up.
- People tell you that you look tired even when you're not.

One of the most often overlooked aspects of the ageing face is the upper third of the face that starts at the level of the eyebrows to the natural hairline. The formula for attractive youthful eyes consists of smooth skin around the eyelids, no fat bulging and eyebrows at or slightly above the rim. No discussion of eyelid rejuvenation would be complete without including the skin of the brow area that also contributes to the eyelids, and vice versa. 'When patients complain that their upper eyelids are sagging, it may be due to drooping of the brow and not the eyelid itself,' says Mr Barry Jones, Past President of the British Association of Aesthetic Plastic Surgeons, adding, 'The ability to lift the brow endoscopically and so not leave a large scar like an Alice band has made a huge difference to facial aesthetic surgery.'

The extent and longevity of brow rejuvenation surgery is variable. The browlift involves repositioning the forehead along with the eyebrows and tissues around the eyes, and reducing furrows between the eyebrows. The result is a more refreshed and open appearance with less crowding around the eyes. The traditional method is the 'open' procedure, which involves repositioning and removing excess skin through an incision that goes across the scalp from a point above the ear and is then closed with sutures or staples. The conventional browlift (also called a coronal lift) has been virtually abandoned by many surgeons who favour the less invasive endoscopic approach (explained in the Keyhole section following). If you already have a high hairline or thinning hair and are concerned about your hairline moving back, beware the browlift. The hairline will be moved back, although considerably less with an endoscopic procedure in which excess skin is not removed. Another technique for the brow area utilizes an incision placed along the hairline (called 'subciliary' in doc speak) to lower the hairline.

Women who are opposed to having a browlift are usually responding to a badly exaggerated result they have seen in someone else. 'I don't want to look surprised,' is a common quip. The eyebrows can sometimes look slightly high immediately following surgery, but most surgeons will tell you that they will settle down as the swelling resolves. If you are indecisive about whether to have a browlift or frightened by the concept of it, you might wind up returning a year later to have it done. If you really need a browlift, having your upper lids done instead will often not achieve your goal, and in fact may actually pull your brows down more. It is imperative that you discuss your eyebrows along with your upper eyelids in consultation with a cosmetic surgeon, as altering one of these areas will ultimately affect the other. If you have determined that you would rather live with your deep forehead creases and droop than opt for surgical intervention, check yourself into the best hair salon you can get and ask for a fringe.

Traditional eyelid surgery

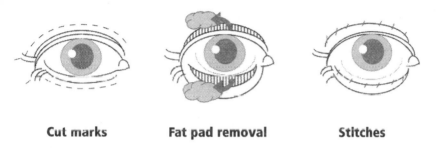

Cut marks **Fat pad removal** **Stitches**

In traditional upper lid rejuvenation, carefully concealed incisions are made in the creases of the upper lid and excess skin and/or fat and/or muscle is removed. Eyelid scars heal well because of the thinness of the skin and they rarely keloid (form excess scar tissue, providing a bobbly effect).

The least invasive surgery for eyelids is the 'transconjunctival' approach of eliminating fatty tissue from the inside of the lid, while maintaining the eyelid's supporting structures. This technique can be applied to the lower as well as upper eyelid fat compartments. Transconjunctival fat removal is typically combined with laser resurfacing to shrink the skin and soften lines and pigment. Lasers are used in two different ways in eyelid surgery: for resurfacing wrinkles and instead of a scalpel. A laser may also be used as a cutting tool in a 'transconjunctival blepharoplasty' procedure. It can be accomplished using a Carbon Dioxide laser to make the incision inside the lid next to where the fat is to be removed. According to Basim Matti, FRCS, 'The lower eyelid is one of the most difficult surgeries. It is safer to be conservative about removing fat and muscle.'

Quiz for aged lids

Snap Test – A clever name for a simple manipulation that indicates whether your eyelid skin has enough zing left. Pinch the eyelid skin, and see if it 'snaps' back into position, or just lingers there limply.

Schirmer Test – If you are having trouble with dry eyes, work out how long you can wear your contact lenses. If the answer is 6–10 hours, you should be fine. If it is less or there are other symptoms of dryness, then a Schirmer test may be a wise precaution to determine if your tear production is up to snuff.

Surgeons approach the fat around the eyelids by preserving it, redistributing it, adding to it or removing it. If the skin is slack, some form of eyelid tightening procedure is needed that will involve removing excess skin and or muscle. According to Dr Bryan Mendelson, FRSCE, FRACS, FACS, 'The lower eyelid is a neutral part of the face compared with the upper lid which can have a significant impact on creating the impression of the personality of the person within. Historically, the treatment of lower lids was to remove all of the protruding fat and then to tighten the skin (and possibly muscle) of the lower lid. Over-resecting the fat can add to an ageing appearance.' If you have sunken hollowing around the eyelids, having all of the fat removed will accentuate that look and increase the chances of wrinkling and other irregularities. Lower eyelids in need of rejuvenation frequently accompany a drooping or sagging of the middle cheeks. The lower lid is connected to the top part of the cheek. When you are in your 20s and early 30s, the soft tissues of the cheek sit high up on the cheekbone. As the years go by, the ageing changes of the lower lid are also manifested in the downward slope of the cheek fat that reveal the bony orbital rims.

The area referred to as the 'mid face', has long been considered to be the most difficult to rejuvenate. A variety of 'cheeklift' or 'mid-facelift' techniques have been developed to reposition your falling fat back up to where it used to be, reduce cheek or 'malar' bags (pouches of skin and fat), and soften the nasal labial folds (those creases that run from the nose to the corners of the mouth). Replacing volume and softness either by grafting or injecting fat or moving your existing fat around can restore a smoother and younger look. Lifting the cheeks is sometimes accomplished through a traditional lower eyelid incision (in the lash line – which has been known to cause the lower eyelid to be pulled down); done endoscopically through incisions in the hairline; and occasionally through incisions inside the mouth. It is an ideal procedure for early ageing changes where the neck is still good, and can be combined with lower facelifting on older women who need more.

keyhole surgery and other modern miracles

The endoscope has become as much a mainstay in the cosmetic surgeon's operating theatre as a microwave in the average kitchen. The applications of endoscopy have expanded considerably since the first time an endoscope was used in cosmetic surgery in 1989. A recent study conducted to review the development of endoscopic techniques in aesthetic and plastic surgery during the last 10 years in the US, Europe and Japan showed impressive results of a 91% reduction in scarring. There is little doubt that the best candidates for minimally invasive endoscopic procedures are in their 30s and early 40s when there is less work to be done.

While endoscopic aesthetic surgery is not literally 'scarless', it certainly minimizes visible scarring. Most endoscopic procedures involve freeing the tissues from their bony attachments and then repositioning them, rather than removing skin or muscle. The endoscopic technique allows surgeons to visualize the inside of the body through a flexible tube with a camera and a light attached to its end. As a natural part of the healing process, the tissues reattach themselves to the bony structures in their new 'lifted' position. Endoscopic techniques can sometimes be combined with conventional or 'open' techniques if you are not a good candidate for purely endoscopic procedures, for example if you've got too much loose skin and excess fat.

Endoscopic browlift

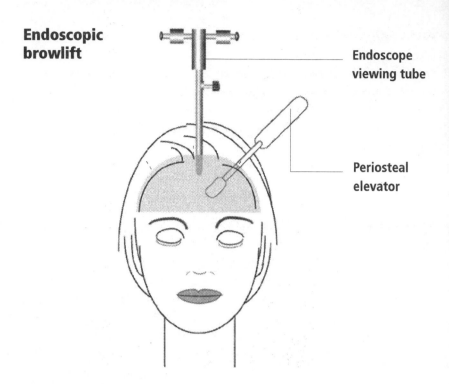

Endoscope viewing tube

Periosteal elevator

The most common aesthetic application of endoscopic instrument-ation is the browlift, a brilliant procedure to resect the muscles that cause frown lines. Several short vertical incisions (3, 4 or 5) within the hairline are all that is needed to do it. The forehead tissues are separated from the skull and then reattached at a higher level using a periosteal elevator. There has been a marked increase in endoscopic techniques in browlifting over the past 6 years due to its many advantages – less scarring and swelling, reduced numbness, less hair loss, less risk of blood clots, and the fact that women prefer it to older methods. The use of the endoscope has changed browlifting from a big procedure with added risks into a technique that even younger women are happy to undergo due to the smaller scars.

The method has evolved dramatically since its introduction in the mid-1990s and innovative surgeons are continuously adjusting their techniques for fixing the brow in its place with dissolvable suturing, staples and screws tunnelled into bone.

Brow rejuvenation

Least invasive	BOTOX
More invasive	Muscle resection (muscles only)
	Browpexy
	Endoscopic browlift (no skin removed)
Most invasive	Open coronal lift (skin + muscle)

The endoscopic technique has its limitations according to Consultant Plastic Surgeon Brian Coghlan, 'It is not suitable for everybody. It is ideal for women who have a crowding of the eyelid area and marked ptosis, and in women who have very active muscles between the brows.' It does not work as well for horizontal forehead lines, which are more commonly treated with BOTOX or laser resurfacing. As Mr Coghlan points out, 'The lift is on the deep layers so you don't necessarily stretch the skin enough to soften all the lines, but you can use BOTOX to extend the results of the browlift and most patients are happy with that.' Although the endoscopic browlift may not be as permanent as an open browlift, you can always have it done again down the line if you need it. Many surgeons world-wide now rarely use the traditional open or coronal incision for browlifting. As Dr Guy Jost describes, 'It is like killing a flea with a bazooka.'

The brow and eyelid area present many variations of clever, inventive techniques. The 'browpexy' utilizes an incision in the upper eyelid crease to lift the eyebrows and fix them to the deeper tissues. This method of minimally invasive brow suspension is good for someone who doesn't want to undergo more complex facial rejuvenation procedures. Another version, the brow suspension technique, secures the eyebrow in this position via two small incisions that are placed over the flat part of the eyebrow, and sometimes with the benefits of incisions placed in the hairline. The access is trickier and the forehead lines will not be smoothed out much with this technique, but it is a good alternative for a woman who is adamant about avoiding an incision in her hairline. Another method to sever the muscles (the corrugators and procerus) that allow you to frown and grimace is called a 'corrugator resection'. This technique strikes a good balance between the short-term effects of BOTOX, and the more long-term improvement from a browlift operation. Small incisions in the crease of the upper eyelid or in the hairline are used to expose the muscles on the area between the eyebrows, which are then separated from the surrounding tissues and removed. The thinning out of these muscles will substantially weaken your ability to create the vertical lines and furrows in the glabellar area between the brows. According to Dr Z. Paul Lorenc, 'Unlike BOTOX, it does not completely paralyse the area and you will still be able to express your emotions. Because not all the muscle fibres can be removed, the result is not entirely permanent, but can easily be repeated in several years' time if needed or treated with BOTOX when muscle activity returns'.

Next, there is the more variable endoscopic facelift. The best candidates are women in their mid-30s to late-40s who are experiencing only the earliest signs of ageing. The operation may involve lifting of the upper and middle face and/or the lower face and neck, as well as a complete facial rejuvenation procedure. With endoscopic surgery, it is possible to reposition the deep, supporting layers to recontour the shape of the face and tone the overlying skin without removing any excess skin. As Dr Foad Nahai explains, 'The endoscopic technique is particularly useful for the younger woman in whom the trade-off of minimal scars v. having some excess skin left is still worthwhile. The role of endoscopy in facelifting continues to evolve and, once the pendulum settles, there is little doubt that it will be firmly integrated into the practice of aesthetic surgery.'

the myths of mini lifts, nips & tucks

Mini is a prefix for useful tools of womanhood like 'skirt', 'bar' and 'series', as well as the name of Mickey's significant other. When followed by 'lift' or 'tuck', 'mini' is one of the true vagaries of cosmetic surgery because it is subject to wide interpretation. A 'mini' means different things to different surgeons as well as to their patients. The trap to avoid is the sort of skin tuck that has been popularized by clinic doctors who have no formal training in surgery of the head and neck. In their hands, all they can do is pull some loose skin from side to side, and tack it up somewhere behind the ear. Just tightening the skin is a futile task. It will not last well because it fails to address the ageing layers underneath. As Mr Norman Waterhouse points out, 'The skin is the least important component of a facelift operation'. 'Mini' has come to refer to something bigger than liposuction of the neck and smaller than a facelift. It is easy to become stuck in the mire of terminology. There is a difference between 'mini' and 'modified'. What remains uncertain is what value 'mini' procedures have. 'Mini' simply means less, whereas, 'modified' indicates that the operation has been tailored to be less invasive while still effective. There are those who find comfort in the concept of lesser surgery. 'I'm not having a facelift, it's just a mini-tuck...' There is less guilt over the sheer vanity of it, and it can't be construed as an admission of having reached 'a certain age' because it's not the real thing. By virtue of those four little letters, the anxiety level of pre-facelift jitters may be dramatically reduced. But even 'minis' come with incisions, anaesthesia, bruising and risks, and are not free unless you happen to be going out with a cosmetic surgeon.

Case history
Louisa Collins, 61, was going through a rough spot in her marriage of 34 years. She had often thought about doing something to get rid of her wobbly neck, but could never quite get up the nerve. Her sister in Glasgow cut out an advert from a cosmetic surgery clinic that showed the

befores and afters of a woman with a big, thick neck who had liposuction. This was just what Louisa was looking for. Although her skin was hanging down and she had a thin, narrow face, the doctor said that liposuction would give her a younger looking neck without scars or surgery and it would cost half the price of a facelift, so she had it done. Several weeks after the surgery, her neck was uneven and the skin was hanging even worse than before surgery. Instead of looking younger, her neck was much droopier and she became clinically depressed. Six months later, Louisa's husband left because he was put off by his wife looking sad and sullen all the time. At the urging of her sister, who felt responsible, Louisa went to see a consultant plastic surgeon in London who told her that the only way to tighten up her neck was with a full facelift, which she should have had in the first place.

Mini factors
Small reasons to consider 'mini' procedures:
- You don't scar well.
- Can't afford the works.
- You are on the young side with less to do.
- Can't take much time off to recover.
- Need it done straight away for a big event.

Shortcut surgeries tend to make me leery, unless there is a good reason to do them and the operation is well thought out. Not everyone is a really good candidate for a 'mini-lift'. In the end, the only thing you may have spared yourself is a long-lasting result. Happiness in mini-lifting and tucking is dependent on working out whether a modified procedure will give you enough change to make it worth your while. As Dr Morrison in Cape Town puts it, 'There is sometimes a law of diminishing returns. A mini operation may give a mini result both in terms of overall effect and also durability of the result. Despite all the wonderful advances in medicine, we will probably never be able to eliminate conventional surgery completely.' The biggest caveat is that mini procedures rarely yield maxi results.

Ms Lena C Andersson
Consultant Plastic Surgeon, Anelca Clinic

- **Are you starting to see women younger and younger?**
  They used to be around 38 or 40-ish, but now we see them earlier for skin fillers and BOTOX from 25 and upwards. Women have become more aware that they can get help with what bothers them at an earlier stage.
- **What do you do to stay ahead of lines and wrinkles?**
  I take plenty of exercise, I don't smoke and I eat healthily. I've had Restylane injected into my worry lines in the glabellar area. I will definitely have something done in the future – the eyelids will be the first for me.
- **What skincare and makeup advice to give your patients?**
  I think a lot of women start using moisturizers too early and they buy cheap formulas. Once a week, it's also good just to do nothing to your skin at all and let it breathe.

Josephine Fairley comes clean about her personal strategy for Feeling Fabulous Forever...
My personal anti-ageing strategy is very much a two-way approach. I believe in taking lots of vitamins and minerals – including a multi antioxidant, vitamin B, lysine (for good, strong skin), and the skin supplement Imedeen and Udo's Choice – an Essential Fatty Acid blend. When I don't take Imedeen and get my EFAs, my skin is more papery. I eat lots of oily fish and plenty of avocados to keep my skin lubricated from the inside-out. I drink, literally, litres of water a day – although I'm not precious about caffeine in tea form. I do yoga and Pilates when I can. I really don't mind being crinkled, but I don't want to be creaky.

Simple is best. Trying lots of anti-ageing products has left me with a legacy of super sensitivity, as I believe many of them have harsh ingredients in order to attain visible benefits. My personal solution is to use facial oils at night, with good, vigorous massage to get the blood flowing. (I don't believe in mollycoddling skin!) And – of course I keep my face out of the sun whenever I can, and wear an SPF15 minimum when I can't.

My favourite beauty treatment is the Rose Body Cocoon at Space NK using aromatherapy oils. Afterwards life feels like it's worth living again and I don't fret so much about anything, let alone lines. I don't worry too much about ageing. I intend to be a FABULOUS and eccentric old woman!

6

two feet...

After 40, a woman has to choose between losing her figure or her face. My advice is to keep your face, and stay sitting down

Dame Barbara Cartland

Ageing is not a uniform experience, but rather an intensely personal phenomenon. Few of us are thoroughly enthralled with the face with which we were born. If you are, then consider yourself part of a rare group. After 35, your face and neck have a mind of their own and the next sound you hear will be your chin plunging at the speed of light and the bags under your eyes going south. At some point in the not-too-distant future, having a little fat injected or the occasional laser peel will no longer be sufficient.

The trend in the UK is advancing rapidly to embrace facial rejuvenation techniques. Reportedly, over 100,000 cosmetic surgical procedures are performed each year and, of those, upwards of 10 % are to the face and eyelids. Professor David Sharpe, OBE, estimates that approximately 5,000 eyelid procedures and 5,000 facelifts are carried out each year and the number is rising steadily. Similarly, according to the Australasian Society of Plastic Surgeons, when their national office was set up in Sydney in 1994, they received approximately 100 enquiries for cosmetic surgery each week. They now average between 50 and 100 enquiries per day.

Facelift facts

The 3 most frequently cited reasons for having a lift:
1. Looking younger.
2. Self-improvement.
3. Facial enhancement.

The 3 top trends noted:
1. Increase in interest in endoscopic surgery.
2. Patients seem more cautious and request less dramatic surgery.
3. Concern about skincare and skin products.

The 4 top increases noted by nearly three-quarters of surgeons:
1. Facelifts.
2. BOTOX.
3. Lip augmentation.
4. Eyelid surgery.

(SOURCE: 1999 survey by Wirthlin Worldwide for the American Academy of Facial Plastic and Reconstructive Surgery)

According to Plastic Surgeon Mr Foad Nahai, 'No two faces age alike and all the anatomical components of facial ageing do not change at exactly the same pace. Reversal of facial ageing is not achieved through surgical rearrangement of the deep tissues and skin excision alone.

Facelift procedures are constantly changing. The facelift I do today bears no resemblance to the first facelift I witnessed in my training many years ago, and very little resemblance to the facelift that I did only a few years ago. As plastic surgeons, we continually work towards improving our results while decreasing the degree of risk.'

the mirror facelift

Every woman over the age of about 35 looks in the mirror, and whether consciously or subconsciously, pulls things up to where they used to be and wishes they could stay there forever. This is known in cosmetic surgery circles as 'the mirror facelift'. If only it was that simple, no woman alive would walk around with saggy jowls. You look at yourself in the mirror and it seems as though the wax is beginning to melt. The critical thing to keep in mind is that the mirror only shows you what you want to see. The universal fallacy of the mirror facelift is that most women place their fingertips right about where the cheekbone ends in the apple of their cheeks and pull sideways as if the skin is caught on a meat hook (see illustration below). The direction of the pull (called the 'vector' in doc speak) is totally unnatural and distorts the features into an alien being.

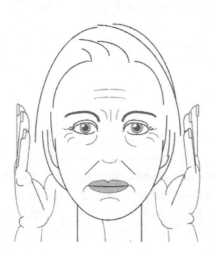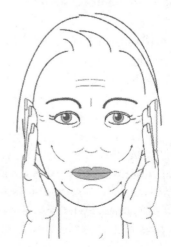

The overriding fear of women on both sides of The Pond is being given the dreaded 'wind tunnel' look, yet fiddling in the mirror with your skin in this manner will produce just that. Your skin and tissues are not stretched so tightly during cosmetic surgery that your circulation is cut off. Instead, they are gently lifted and stitched into place in layers. If your surgeon yanked you straight back towards your ears, your mouth would widen and your scars would stretch. As Dr Bernard Cornette de Saint Cyr explains, 'The actual concept of facial rejuvenation surgery is face remodelling, not face pulling.'

Mirror, mirror

Have you ever imagined what you would look like after a lift? You can emulate how the skin and muscles are redraped by doing these two simple exercises. The first exercise shows you your skin folds; the second shows you how you will look when the face has been lifted.

Before lift

1. Sit in a chair.
2. Place a hand mirror on your lap.
3. Look straight down.
4. Note the folds in your skin.

After lift

1. Lie on your bed.
2. Hold the hand mirror over your face.
3. Look up (if your bedroom ceiling is mirrored, skip number 2).
4. Note the natural lift of your skin.

Think of the mirror as an essential beauty tool, an aid to self-discovery. Study the variations in your face, the curves, contours and marks of distinction. Note any asymmetries from right to left. No face is identical on both sides, and invariably upon investigation you will note that one brow is lower than the other or one eye smaller. Pull out your family photograph album to contrast the face you now have to the one you had formerly. Surgeons will often encourage patients to bring in a photo of themselves at the mark of a decade, for example at age 30, 40, 50, and so on. This is not to suggest that you can reasonably assume that you will look exactly like that again, but it is a great indicator of what liberties the ageing process has taken with your face.

Resist the temptation to compare yourself to celebrities. It is grossly unfair and can be an instant downer. Pop stars, footballers, supermodels, It-girls and film divas look and live in a state of permanent luxe that mere mortals can never come close to. They thrive in the intense scrutiny of the public eye that necessitates being all glammed up and ready for a close-up on a daily basis. A mother of three in the counties, whose days are spent in denims and wellies tidying up the garden, cannot be expected to compete with Liz Hurley slithering about in Versace after hours of preening and pampering.

The older you get, the more you recognize the shortage of natural beauties there are in the world. Celebrities are gorgeous because they are presented to us as pure fantasy. A magazine cover featuring a head shot of Mrs Crawford from Kent in a tweed suit from M&S wouldn't sell nearly as well as a half-naked Kate Moss draped in Calvin. The great injustice is that many celebrities swear that they haven't had a spot of 'work' done when they most definitely have. It sets up an unrealistic standard for all the Mrs Crawfords in the world that is deceptive and misleading. Mrs Crawford has only to compare her 60-something face with that of Sophia Loren and she will undoubtedly wonder where she has gone wrong and curse nature for failing her.

Looking great is not necessarily synonymous with perfection. Even the ultimate beauties of our time have their share of wrinkles. It just isn't realistic for any woman over 18 to have a flawless face, except via the benefit of serious re-touching.

For women whose entire identity is based solely on how they look, there is a natural, built-in predisposition to high anxiety at the thought of losing that. If you majored in being beautiful from a young girl up through your 30s, your 40s will be difficult to accept. None of us are actually happy with the signs of age, but most of us don't make a hobby out of grieving for the loss of our young faces. The only person who will dissect every line and mark is you, as everyone else is much more concerned with his or her own lines and marks. The key is to be proactive instead of reactive; learn to make your best features work for you and take care of the lines before they take over.

Amanda Lacey, 30-something London facialist, on the uniqueness of ageing:
On surgical intervention, one should be selective and approach it with care as surgery can change the individual characteristics that are unique. I hope that by the time I consider intervention, methods will have become more non-invasive.

too early v. too late

The ideal age to have a facelift is when you think you need one. Some women are sure they need a lift when they really don't. Other women are convinced they don't need a facelift yet or they're not ready, when, in fact, they are overdue. I make it a habit never to respond to women who query me with, 'How old do you think I look?' There is no good response to a loaded question like that, and it is a double-edged sword whether your guesstimate is higher or lower than the correct number. Women place far too much emphasis on being a certain age, and basing the need for a facelift merely on a big birthday is oversimplifying the decision.

Once the bastion of silver-haired women in their middle to late 50s, the facelift continues to gain popularity among women in their early 40s. If you're in your 40s and your face is showing signs of ageing, opting for a facelift early instead of waiting has its advantages. 'Since the surgeon is usually dealing with better-quality tissues in patients in their 40s, the results look better and last longer,' says Dr Donald Wood-Smith, adding, 'The bottom line is that a woman who has a facelift at 45 is generally going to have the edge over someone who has her first facelift in her 50s.'

Am I ready for a facelift?

Some of the signals that you may be inching your way towards the 'F' word are a slackening up along the jawline, neck and cheeks. Check off all that apply:

- Everyone around you looks younger than you do.
- You can no longer locate the bones of your jawline.
- You avoid having your picture taken.
- You never want to be on top any more.
- You find yourself using the back of your hand to support your chin.
- You reapply your powder and foundation several times a day.
- No price is too high to pay for a cream that 'firms'.
- Every day is a bad hair day and you're constantly reinventing your hairstyle.
- You switch from mock to turtlenecks.
- Friends start saying 'it makes you look younger…'
- You speed up as you pass shop windows, in case you see your reflection.
- You get misty eyed when you see old photographs of yourself.
- You switch from 'regular' to 'extra strength' everything.
- You bought this book for yourself and you're holding on to it for dear life.

If one part of the face is ageing and out of sync with the rest of the face which still looks good, you could have a localized procedure to bring the face back into balance. According to Basim A. Matti, FRCS, 'Women are coming in at age 30 to 35 for BOTOX around the eyes and the glabellar and then they progress to eyelid surgery with or without the endoscopic browlift. The introduction of BOTOX has greatly reduced the number of browlifts we do.'

Some women are simply not ready for a facelift in their 40s for a variety of reasons. There are definite pitfalls of doing too much surgery too early. One that springs to mind is that you may start to actually look older. Obviously lifted and pulled faces tend to make people think you must be centuries older than you really are and have the scars to prove it. Another factor is the self-limiting aspects of premature plastic surgery. Any procedure that in any way limits your future options should be given careful consideration before diving in. These would include anything that creates a visible scar and scar tissue that may interfere with additional procedures later on.

The advantages of an early lift

- Leads to a better result.
- Lasts longer.
- Short recovery.
- Does not preclude a full facelift later on.
- Maintains skin structure.

The face is said to age the fastest between the ages of 40 and 45. Women whose faces are not ageing evenly must decide whether a localized procedure such as just doing the eyelids should be done now or whether they would be better served by waiting a year or two to have a total rejuvenation. The works might include a forehead lift, eyelid surgery, a face- and neck-lift with some laser resurfacing, which would qualify as 'the gold standard' of facial rejuvenation. Mr Brian Coghlan explains that women fall loosely into three distinct groups. The first group are in their late 30s and early 40s and are looking into having a facelift, but may not need it yet. They may choose to do fat transfer instead to stave off the lift for a few more years. The second group are in their mid- to late-40s and are candidates for their first lift, which may only be a modified or endoscopically-assisted mid-facelift or temporal lift. The third group are women in their late 50s and 60s who are only planning to have one facelift and want to get as much of a difference out of it as they can.

One of the disadvantages of putting it off is that if you wait until your face is falling, the after-effects will be more obvious to everyone. The more work there is to do, the more dramatically different you will look when it's all done. Another disadvantage is that you have a chance to get a better result on more elastic tissues. In some cases, you may be happier to tackle all the problems in the face at once because the better result produces an endless ripple effect. Otherwise, 6 months later the only thing you'll be able to see is that tiny imperfection you failed to address. For example, the woman who is on the fence about 'to browlift or not to browlift' almost always regrets not having done it later on and joins the ranks of other BOTOX junkies.

It is never really too late to have your first facelift, as long as you are in good health and your doctor is reasonably certain that you can survive the surgery. There are women who wait to have their eyelids or face lifted as late as their mid-70s, although it is not the norm. Recovering from the effects of surgery and an anaesthetic takes longer at that age, and the process is more of a physical and emotional ordeal. It is more common to have a first facelift in your 50s or 60s, and a more minor secondary procedure later on in life. According to the American College of Surgeons, 'The first report of a surgical procedure being performed on someone over the age of 100 was in 1985'. At the beginning of the 20th century, life expectancy was 49, but today it is a mighty 82. At the rate of advancements in modern surgical and anaesthetic techniques, older patients are becoming suitable candidates for facial rejuvenation procedures. I just hope that when I hit 80, I will still care about my wrinkles and my bags. When you stop caring entirely, that would be cause for alarm.

neck lines

Every woman dreams of having a graceful, swanlike neck like Audrey Hepburn or Vivien Leigh, two timeless English beauties that epitomize the engaging femininity of a slender, well-defined jawline. Ageing has a way of smudging the continuous line that runs from the face to the neck, as if the artist's sleeve brushed against his charcoal drawing. Although you might not notice it from the front, the oblique and profile views expose the neck at its scraggiest. To get the full effect, stand in front of the mirror and look down at your Clarks. Yikes! Now you see them, all three of your chins that look remarkably like the neck of a bloodhound. The frequently overlooked ageing neck and décolletage is really an extension of the face and demands the same degree of care. Regrettably, the jawline rarely gets the attention it deserves in terms of moisturizing and sun protection. As the neck has fewer oil glands than other visible areas of the upper body, it is more subject to the ravages of free radicals, neglect and birthdays.

Loosening skin on the neck is a problem of the 40s onwards that affects women struggling with sagging skin and an increase in fatty tissues. Yo-yo dieting is another common culprit. Over 40, losing a stone or two will make your waistline younger, but may also put a few years on your lower face.

Cosmetic surgeons can approach the neck in several ways. The most important factor is to work out whether your ageing neck is related to the skin and/or musculature. On a younger neck, they can vacuum away unwanted fat in the neck and jowl areas using liposuction. The procedure can take as little as 20 minutes and gives the neck a sharper line and better contour. Liposuction alone is brilliant on young, toned skin under 40 or so. However, when just fat is suctioned from an older neck, the underlying muscle bands, hanging glands and loose skin may show up more after the cushiony fatty tissue that was camouflaging these structures is removed. Similarly, neck flaws are easier to spot in a thin neck. On a younger woman with a thick neck and weak chin, sucking out the excess fat can work wonders to recontour the neck and make the chin look more prominent.

The key is in the quality and quantity of the skin. If you have loose skin or a 'turkey gobbler' neck to start with, a bigger procedure is probably indicated. If you don't want a complete facelift, and you have loose skin and bands around your neck, a 'platysmaplasty' may be performed by resewing the muscle bands together through an incision under the neck with a suture suspension technique. A necklift can also be done endoscopically, alone or in addition to other work in the upper face. This method allows for excess fat to be removed that rests above and/or below the muscle in the neck, and/or later tightening of the neck muscles, suspension suture placement, usually without skin removal. If the skin is very slack, a lower facelift will give better control in most patients. According to Mr Alan Matarasso, 'If there is more advanced skin sagging than liposculpting of the jowls and chin can address, there's no replacement for facelift surgery.'

Doing just your neck when your cheeks are drooping as well will create disharmony, according to Consultant Plastic Surgeon Basim A. Matti, FRCS, who prefers to do the face and neck together: 'When combined with more extensive facial rejuvenation, the choice of

facelift technique greatly influences the choice of necklift technique.'
Carol, a nurse from Cheshire, compared it to painting only one wall
of a dreary room. Surgeons have been known to pull out all the stops
to achieve a smooth angle where the neck meets the chin on necks
that have not weathered well.

Save your neck

Problem	Solution
Muscle bands	BOTOX
Neck rings, crêpey skin	BOTOX/anti-ageing skincare
Wrinkles/age spots	Peels/lasers
Fatty tissue	Neck liposuction
Sagging skin, muscles, fat (a little)	Endoscopic necklift or Lower facelift
Sagging skin, muscles, fat (a lot)	Full face- and necklift

For me, the true test of a brilliant lift is how clean and smooth the
resulting jawline is. Many women complain at first that their neck is
stiff, sore and feels as though they are being strangled. As the swelling
comes down, these same women will invariably be measuring every
last soupçon of loose flesh under their chins. Somewhere around the
6-month anniversary, armies of women around the world march en
masse to their plastic surgeons' consulting rooms, pinching more than
an inch of their neck skin to illustrate their dissatisfaction, 'Doctor,
couldn't you have made this a little tighter...?'

the whole hog

Aesthetic surgeons are in the profession of making people look good, or better, as the case may be. The role of the surgeon is to evaluate the face and advise its owner about what will produce the best aesthetic result. The role of the patient, if you will, is to approach the doctor by articulating what bothers her and inquiring, 'what can you do to fix this?' Ultimately, no one can tell you what to do with your face. With the dawn of combination therapies and the increase in the sheer number of options available, more women are having 'facial rejuvenation' procedures than just plain lifts and tucks. Women are learning to look at their faces as a whole unit, beginning at the hairline and ending just above the collarbone, instead of focusing solely on the feature that offends them as they're putting on their makeup.

The three zones of the face

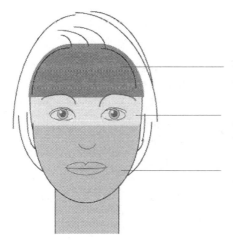

Zone I The forehead area from the eyebrows up to the hairline

Zone II The eyelid region to the cheeks

Zone III The lower face and neck

A facelift operation is concerned primarily with Zones II and III (mid and lower face and neck) and makes only subtle improvements in Zone I (eyes and forehead). According to Mr Barry Jones, 'The vast majority of developments in facial rejuvenation surgery over the last 30 years have arisen out of craniofacial surgery, which in turn has given us a much better understanding of facial anatomy. One can think of the face in layers and rejuvenative techniques which may be applied to each of them – the skin, fascia, fat and muscle, periosteum.'

The 4 basic facelifts

SMAS LIFT
Excess skin is removed and redraped, the skin and the SMAS (underlying muscle layer) are elevated and tightened, and fatty tissue under the neck is suctioned.

EXTENDED SMAS LIFT
Excess skin is removed and redraped, the underlying muscle layer is freed from the cheek ligaments and more tension is placed on the muscle layer instead of the skin flap.

SUBPERIOSTEAL LIFT
Sometimes referred to as the Mask Lift. This procedure can be done with an endoscope and/or via an incision running horizontally across the scalp, with or without incisions placed inside the mouth to free the fat, muscle and skin layers off the bone so they can be pulled up and tightened.

COMPOSITE LIFT
Also called a Deep Plane Facelift, this a total facial rejuvenation including the upper and lower eyelids, an open browlift, face and neck. The facial tissues, fat, muscles and skin are lifted in one continuous section.

In addition to the above variations, there are modified face- and neck-lifts with or without endoscopic assistance, as well as the skin lift or subcutaneous facelift, in which only the skin is redraped. In most cases, an incision is made in the hairline at the temple, extending into the skin creases in front of the ear or behind the tragus (the bit of cartilage that sticks out) of the ear, around the ear lobe and behind the ear, finishing in the hairline of the scalp. If fat under the chin is suctioned and/or the muscles in the neck are tightened, an incision will also be placed under the chin. The incisions must provide enough access for the surgeon to separate skin from the underlying fat and muscles and do his job effectively. The skin is then repositioned upwards and backwards and sideways as needed, and excess skin is removed. Each surgeon has his own exact criteria for choosing where to place the incisions, depending on hairline and bone structure, and will vary the method slightly with every facelift he performs. No two faces are alike, and thus, no two facelifts are alike, either. Women are keen to have the latest procedures if they have been proven to be of good quality, but they don't want to take the risk of a lot of complications. All women want a good result that will last, but the flipside is that not all women are willing to have aggressive surgery.

Deep lifts

According to Dallas Plastic Surgeon Dr Sam Hamra, 'The face ages predictably from the top down and skin first.' The two premises of the 'composite' lift, formerly known as the 'deep plane' facelift, are simple: the facelift tension is pulled in a different direction than standard methods (up, instead of back), and the fat and muscles are repositioned in one unit. The term 'composite' refers to all areas of the face being moved together, i.e. the three zones of the face: the lower face, around the eyes ('periorbital' in doc speak), and the forehead. The neck and brow are always done (low brows are lifted and high foreheads are lowered) along with the face to maintain facial harmony. If your brow area is sagging and it is not corrected at the same time as your face and neck, the top third of your face will effectively end up looking older than the rest. As Dr Hamra explains, 'The mission of the composite lift is to recreate the contours of youth without the stigma of a facelifted look, and/or to restore the youthful contours on a previously lifted face.'

Deeper facelifts tend to be more invasive than conventional methods, and produce more prolonged swelling, so they might put a major crimp in your social calendar for a few months. The stated advantages are a longer-lasting result and a more harmonious appearance. The bigger the job you are having done, the more confidence, experience and in-depth knowledge of underlying facial structures (nerves, muscles, fat pads, veins) are required in your surgeon. According to Dr Bryan Mendelson, 'Deeper procedures are premised on the tightening of the ligamentous support between the SMAS and the facial skeleton so that the result is not overdone. The benefit of the deep plane procedures, when performed properly, is that the patient will have the appearance that they would have had a decade earlier, and this decade of benefit continues throughout life.'

Cosmetic surgeons are doing more facelifts with eyelids and browlifting, along with some version of resurfacing and BOTOX for dynamic wrinkles and fat grafts for lips and deeper folds, all at one stage. A logical place to draw that line is usually where the neck meets the torso. Regrettably, a facelift alone cannot do it all. A chorus of familiar refrains from women leafing through befores and afters includes, 'she should have done her eyes too' to 'what about those lines around her mouth' or the ever-popular, 'I can't tell the difference'. The facelift primarily improves a scraggy neck and jowling. It does not remove wrinkles, fine lines around the mouth and crow's feet and cannot erase natural facial lines of expression like the nasal labial folds that run from the nose to the corners of the mouth.

As Dr Frank Trepsat explains, 'There is something strange about a face that has only one aspect of youth; tightness, but not fullness.' The modern weapons of choice for replacing lost volume are fillers, specifically fat. For wrinkles and skin texture, lasers, dermabraders and peeling solutions provide the finishing touches to a beautiful lift. Having a lift done without paying attention to the condition of your skin is akin to hiring a turf accountant who doesn't use a calculator. If you don't do anything about the little lines around your mouth, they will invariably stand out after everything else is smooth. Although you may understand intellectually that your facelift will not obliterate every line, women secretly wish it were so and hope for the best.

The most common remark about a lifted acquaintance is often, 'She doesn't have a line on her face'. Skin resurfacing is added at the end of a facelift, like the fabric used to reupholster your old living room sofa.

Facelifting and lasers are not interchangeable, and laser resurfacing is no substitute for a facelift. If you are frightened of having surgery, full-face resurfacing with a Carbon Dioxide laser is an infinitely worse experience. In fact, any woman who undergoes both laser resurfacing and a facelift will undoubtedly complain more about the after-effects of the laser.

Modern innovations

- **Tissue glue** – Fibrin-based tissue sealants and adhesives have gained widespread acceptance as versatile surgical tools. Although commercial tissue sealants have been used for many years in Europe, the FDA approval in the United States has stimulated research into cosmetic surgery applications. Made from human and bovine (cow) tissue extracts, tissue glue or Fibrin, sealant is sprayed on to hold tissues in place and accelerate the healing process. According to Dr Peter Bela Fodor, 'The glue is particularly useful for sealing tissues that have been lifted, and reduces swelling and bruising after surgery.'
- **Absorbable sutures** – Coated Vicryl Rapide (Johnson & Johnson) is a rapidly absorbing suture material commonly used in cosmetic surgery. It dissolves in the body within 1–2 weeks and does not require removal.

As Mr Coghlan puts it, 'There is no such thing any more as a "formula facelift". Now we're picking out bits of different procedures that will suit the patient to individualize the lift for her.' Women don't necessarily go to a cosmetic surgeon to have one isolated thing done. They often have several on their own or lumped together. There is certainly room for more than one way to lift an ageing face, and that, as they say, is what makes a horse race. Short of going to medical school, you can't be expected to fully understand the subtleties of SMASectomy v. Extended SMAS v. Platysmaplasty, and so on. Getting bogged down with the hopelessly technical aspects of facelift surgery can be unnecessarily daunting. What one surgeon calls 'subperiosteal', another surgeon will call a 'mask lift', and still a third will execute the same operation via a different plan of incisions entirely. Even if you think you know everything there is to know about facelifting techniques, another one will shortly come along to throw you off.

The right facelift for you is really more about picking a good surgeon, communicating what you want to achieve and passing the job of selecting the best method to the surgeon. The other key is to light a candle at Westminster Abbey. The rest is down to just a little dash of luck.

7

taking the plunge

The days of getting lifted and hiding out in the country manor for a season are long since gone. Women today want to get back to their lives quickly, whether they are chairing a committee, taking their children to school, or running a limited company. Fortunately, sweeping advances in cosmetic surgery technology and instrumentation, together with shorter-acting anaesthetics, means that the recovery process is not only shorter but, in many cases, next to painless.

The real life day-to-day practicalities of having cosmetic surgery – of scheduling, preparing, finding the right 'lift attendants' to manage your recovery, who to tell and what to say, and how and when to stage your first re-entry into public life – all take on paramount importance. One seemingly inconsequential pearl of wisdom from an experienced lift-ee on issues of critical importance, such as hair emergencies, flawless guerrilla camouflage techniques, what to stock up on before and after surgery and how to keep your wits about you, can prove invaluable later on. As the Boy Scouts are fond of saying, always be prepared. Being ready, willing and able takes some of the fear and anxiety out of the process because you will know what to expect and how to handle every eventuality. As idyllic as it may sound to have every body part re-sculpted at the same time, it may be more than you and your surgeon are willing to take on.

cosmetic surgery is not for the weak at heart

Ladies, hold on to your hats. I have to tell you something of vital importance. Cosmetic surgery is not a day at the beach. IT IS REAL SURGERY. As it is elective, it is often performed outside the normal controls imposed on the medical profession by governments and other third parties. The fact that cosmetic surgery is generally done on healthy people, not the elderly or infirm, does not justify any lessening of customary standards of medical care. The longer and more extensive the surgery, the greater the chance of complications. Cosmetic surgery operations, at least in the UK, are typically done in hospital and involve the use of an anaesthetic and, as such, should never be taken lightly.

The pre-operative evaluation
The overriding rule in all areas of medicine is 'Primum non-nocere', or 'Do no harm.' Cosmetic surgery is certainly no exception. According to GP Dr Susan Horsewood-Lee, 'Since cosmetic surgery is elective, there are unfortunately few legal safeguards and it is often performed outside the normal controls imposed on medical specialities. If you have a supportive health professional, ask your GP to do a pre-operative health screening to isolate any contra-indications

that need attention before surgery is contemplated; for example, anaemia, blood clotting problems, positive hepatitis status and other liver problems, diabetes or hypertension. If you are not medically fit for surgery, a responsible cosmetic surgeon will dissuade you from having it.' You will be required to have a routine health screening prior to surgery to assess your general health and condition, often at the hospital where the surgery will be performed.

Pre-surgical screening
- General medical examination.
- Height and weight measurements.
- Blood pressure measurement.
- Urine analysis.
- Blood analysis.
- Chest X-ray.
- Resting electrocardiogram.
- Psychological profile/assessment.

According to Dr Horsewood-Lee, 'Your surgeon will request that you stop smoking, cut down on alcohol, caffeine, aspirin and aspirin-containing drugs, stop taking HRT, contraceptive pills (you may experience an unusual bleeding pattern as a result), and all other medications, including vitamins and minerals, to minimize the risk of blood clots.' She also recommends addressing anxiety and doubts by talking and sharing the experience with someone close to you. Yoga, meditation and self-hypnosis can also be of value. 'Maintaining a fitness regime is helpful right up to surgery, then take a break and resume 2–3 weeks later, depending on the surgery,' she adds.

The day of the operation
For smaller facial procedures, surgery can be arranged as an ambulatory or day case, either in hospital or in your doctor's surgery. In some cases, you might be admitted to the hospital the evening before your operation, which is especially helpful if you live far from

the hospital or clinic. For the majority of facelifts in the UK, you will be admitted to hospital on the day of surgery and will stay overnight. In America, Australia, Canada and other parts of Europe, it is common to have cosmetic procedures done in a clinic or surgery suite and to go home the same day.

You will be instructed on the importance of not eating or drinking anything (that includes water and tea) after midnight on the eve of surgery because of the risk of aspirating the contents of your stomach up into your throat when your muscles are relaxed under anaesthetic, which can cause you to choke. If for any reason you have broken the rules, this is not a time to keep quiet for fear of embarrassment. You MUST notify your anaesthetist or your surgeon.

Case history

A recognizable TV actress of the 1980s was admitted into one of New York's top clinics for a tuck performed by its top surgeon. In an effort to offer gracious hospitality, the clinic sent the actress a lovely basket of fruit the evening before her surgery. The fruit was tempting and the starlet took a large bite out of a ripe banana the night before her op. Her surgery had to be cancelled until it was safe to administer the anaesthetic.

Pre-operative skin markings

Cosmetic surgeons will draw a map of the planned operation on your face. Your surgeon will use a dark purple or blue felt pen to mark exactly where he will be making the incisions. It will not be necessary to shave your scalp or any hair on the skin around the site of the operation. For face and browlifts, the hair is neatly parted and wrapped with tight rubber bands or sterile clips and combs to keep it out of the surgeon's way.

Blood transfusions

Facial cosmetic surgery does not involve a substantial loss of blood and the surgeon is expected to carefully tie off and control bleeding vessels. For this reason, blood transfusions are unnecessary.

the big sleep – anaesthetics

Some women may be as apprehensive (or more so) about having an anaesthetic as they are about the surgery. According to Consultant Anaesthetist Dr Peter Forrester, who specializes in anaesthesia for cosmetic surgery at The Wellington Hospital, 'Modern anaesthesia is safer than it has ever been. This is mainly because of improvements in three key areas: better training and understanding, safer, modern drugs that affect body systems less and that wear off more quickly after surgery, and vastly improved monitoring equipment that allows for a very careful watch on vital body functions.'

Although there is a wide spectrum in the level of anaesthetics, there are two main categories – local and general, with twilight resting in the middle. Methods of blocking pain sensation from specific areas of the face and body have improved so much in recent years that many minor cosmetic procedures can be done using some form of local anaesthetic, with or without sedation.

Local anaesthetics

There is no loss of consciousness with local anaesthesia, so patients are able to communicate with the surgeon. The local anaesthetic agents temporarily prevent the nerves from carrying pain messages to the brain. The injection may be given directly into the area to be operated on, or around the main trunks of the nerves that carry sensation. Another form of local anaesthetic used in cosmetic procedures is a topical or surface form. This is used for all injectable treatments, such as BOTOX, collagen and fat transfer, as well as laser resurfacing. A spray or cream is applied to the area to be numbed – a common sight in fashionable central London consulting rooms is a line up of ladies with thick white, creamy moustaches waiting for their lips to be sufficiently deadened so that they can have their beauty shots.

Twilight sedatives

Cosmetic procedures are often performed under a local anaesthetic with the addition of a 'twilight' sedative given intravenously, such as diazepam (Valium), so you can be thoroughly relaxed. You will be in a sleepy state, but may drift in and out of consciousness. This allows the area being operated on to be numbed, while you are relaxed but not as heavily sedated as you would be with a general anaesthetic.

General anaesthetics

A general anaesthetic is commonly used in larger surgical procedures, such as a full facelift with eyelids and browlift, where the body is going to sustain a substantial amount of trauma. A general anaesthetic is administered by injection, gas, or a combination of both, and causes you to fall into a deep sleep. Other non-anaesthetic drugs are used to take away all sensations, to relax your muscles, and to keep you from going into shock. The anaesthetist puts you to sleep (if you are not already asleep from the pre-operative injection) by giving you a small injection of rapidly acting and powerful drugs. Modern anaesthetics work so quickly and efficiently that, as soon as your IV drip goes in, it will seem to you that you are waking up in the recovery room, astonished to find it is all over and asking what the time is.

The anaesthetist

The final clearance before surgery actually rests in the hands of the anaesthetist who will visit you on the morning of the operation to ensure that you are fit for surgery and that the anaesthetic is going to be safe. If your blood pressure is elevated or you have a chest infection or are running a slight fever, your surgery is likely to be cancelled or postponed until you are well. This is the time to divulge any shoulder, back or neck problems you may have as well, so he can position your body appropriately during the surgery. If you suffer from any excessive fears or anxiety disorders such as claustrophobia, now is the time to speak up.

What you will be asked

- If there is any chance you could be pregnant or if you are breast-feeding.
- The date of your last menstrual period.
- What medications you are currently taking.

- If you have had any previous reactions to an anaesthetic.
- If you have any allergies to medications.
- If you are a smoker.
- When you last ate or drank.

Premedication

Your will usually have a chance to talk with your surgeon and ask any last-minute questions before you are given any medications. The anaesthetist will ask if you want to be sleepy and relaxed before surgery. Some people much prefer to be fully awake and in control right up to induction of anaesthesia. Premeds can be the antidote to having the urge to break loose and cut a path down the hospital corridor to freedom, knocking over a few nurses as you go. If you are particularly jittery about the surgery, the warm, relaxing sensation of a sedative can do wonders for your state of mind as the time for the operation draws nearer. It is also quite normal to have anxiety and get cold feet as you try to fall asleep the night before your facelift. If you think you will need a sedative the night before surgery, your GP might give you a prescription for a single dose. Even when you may have total confidence in your surgeon, when it is your face he is operating on, you are destined to worry.

The operating theatre

Once you are wheeled into the operating theatre, the anaesthetist will begin by giving you a small injection that will make you feel drowsy. Within seconds you will be completely unconscious, and that is usually the last thing you will remember of the actual procedure. If you will be under anaesthetic for several hours, you may have a rubber or plastic tube called a catheter inserted inside the urethra and into the bladder to keep it empty during the surgery. Your anaesthetic will be supplied continuously to keep you comfortably asleep during the operation while a pulse oximeter, a small device clipped onto your fingertip, will monitor your heart rate, ECG tracing, blood pressure, breathing rate and the volume of gases you are breathing by the minute.

'The modern monitoring equipment we use continuously checks the patient's condition, and especially the level of oxygen in the blood, and provides more reliable surveillance than ever before,' says Dr Forrester, adding, 'the crucial thing is that modern monitoring allows us to detect and correct little problems at an earlier stage than previously, before they turn into big problems.' If you are concerned that you might reveal your most intimate secrets under the effects of the anaesthetic, no one will be taking notes or recording you. If you are having only light sedation, it is possible to mumble some words during surgery, but with general anaesthesia you are in a very deep sleep. If you are able to carry on a conversation or move about, it will signal to the anaesthetist that you need a larger dose of medications to keep you well sedated. You will have no recollection of being conscious or feeling any pain.

Waking up

Once you are stable and feeling reasonably comfortable and clear-headed, you can be discharged into the care of a responsible adult if you are a day case, or wheeled back into your room if you are staying in hospital. One of the things that can cause bleeding and haematoma (blood clotting around the wound site) is the patient getting up too soon. The best thing after a facelift is to spend the first 4–6 hours dozing. You will feel lightly sleepy and pleasantly groggy. As Dr Forrester says, 'The patients that are standing on the balcony when I walk into the room are the ones that frighten me.'

With today's modern short-acting drugs, you may feel like getting up and about within a few hours of the last few stitches being tied off, but you'll have less swelling and bruising if you get proper rest immediately following surgery. The first 12 hours are the most critical for post-operative complications. The risk of haematoma or bleeding declines within the first 24 hours, and continues to decline up to a week, when it levels off. Haematoma can be caused by straining, sitting on the toilet, bending over or exerting yourself too soon (and that includes having sex). Small amounts of the anaesthetic drugs will remain in your body for up to 24 hours after the operation. Although you may feel wide-awake, you will still be under the influence of these medications during this period. Your concentration and co-ordination may be impaired and you may suddenly feel lightheaded or faint. You will be instructed not to make any important decisions, like who to leave your jewels to, and not to operate heavy machinery. Trust me, the last thing on your mind right after a facelift will be getting yourself up to plough your acres.

Antibiotics

There is a concern among the medical community that a growing number of germs have become resistant to antibiotics. Many common infections are now impervious to formerly reliable drugs. The more often an antibiotic is used, the more likely it is that bacteria will become resistant to it. Therefore, surgeons today have cut down on their precautionary use of antibiotics in cosmetic surgery. Your doctor will prescribe antibiotics if necessary, sometimes starting before and/or continuing after the lift to prevent infection. Keflex is commonly used and your anaesthetist will usually give you a dose of antibiotic in your intravenous fluids as well during surgery.

Pain relief

The anaesthetic will contain painkillers so that you will not be too uncomfortable when you first wake up. As soon as the anaesthetic begins to wear off, the nurses will give you further painkillers, which may be in the form of tablets or injections. You will also routinely be given some painkillers to take home with you. According to Dr Forrester, 'A facelift is a remarkably painless operation and most women need only paracetamol or a mild codeine mixture. With an endoscopic browlift, about half the patients will have a bad headache for the first 12 hours, which may require an injection of morphine.' You may find it helpful to take painkillers before going to sleep at night to relax you. If you are not used to taking medications, painkillers may cause side effects, such as lightheadedness, dizziness, drowsiness, nausea, constipation or sickness. 'True allergy to codeine and the other opiates is quite uncommon; when most patients say that they are allergic to codeine and other painkilling drugs, it usually means that it makes them feel nauseated,' says Dr Forrester. If you can't tolerate the recommended dosage, you can try reducing the dose from two to one tablet or switch to plain paracetamol instead. Most facelift patients will not need to take pain medications after the first few days.

Nausea

If you have a history of being nauseated from medications or motion sickness, you may be sick from your anaesthetic and/or pain medication. You should alert your anaesthetist if you have a tendency to get nauseated from drugs and he will give you an anti-emetic in your IV drip during surgery. With today's modern anaesthetics, the incidence of nausea has been greatly reduced. If you do get sick, regrettably, it is often what you remember most about your facelift experience, and it can be very unpleasant. I can recall many late nights spent handing a patient a stainless steel bowl and waiting outside the bathroom door, hoping she didn't pop a suture loose while heaving.

Supporting pillows

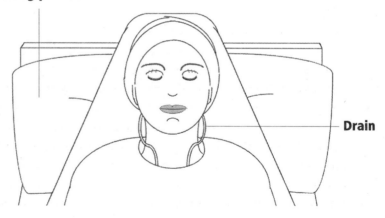

Drain

Dressings

Depending on how much lifting and tucking you've had, you may go home with some bandages still on. Dressings range from a few simple steri-strips for a neck that has been liposuctioned and an elastic strap or band stretched around your head, to a gauzy facelift netting and a soft plastic drain poking out from behind each ear. There will be varying types of sutures, some that have to be removed and others that will dissolve on their own in about a week, plus 'clips' or surgical staples that may be used in the hair-bearing parts of the scalp. You should expect some formal instructions on what to take off when, which to keep dry, and when to change soiled pads.

The trip home

Like wine, a newly lifted face does not travel well. If you are planning a long journey home after surgery, think again. Up to two hours is manageable, but any longer may be risky, especially if you are prone to motion sickness. Whenever possible, stay close to the clinic or hospital, or preferably in it for that matter. Never go home by yourself after having anaesthesia. Arrange to have an adult companion, friend or family member take you home and stay with you for the first 24 hours to help you get settled. You'll need to schedule at least one follow-up appointment so that the doctor will be able to check the healing of your incisions and for his nurse to remove dressings and sutures. Don't expect your surgeon to take out your sutures. It is common practice to leave matters of stitches to nursing staff, who are usually more benevolent and light-handed about it, anyway.

Case history

Elaine and Beverly Stringer, two sisters in their middle 60s, were living on their family estate in a rural town. Elaine was recommended to a plastic surgeon an hour away for her to have her deviated septum (nose) fixed and to ask about some cosmetic work. As they were both retired and had some extra money to spend on themselves, Beverly decided to have a tummy tuck and a facelift as well. Elaine decided to let Beverly go first and she would take care of her. Beverly's surgery was carried out in the doctor's clinic and took 5 hours under a general anaesthetic. Although she wasn't feeling all that well while she was in recovery, the surgery had been scheduled as a day case and the plan was for Elaine to drive her back home for the night. Neither the doctors nor the nursing staff suggested that perhaps Beverly should stay the night or have surgery in hospital or arrange a private nurse for her. Her trip home was miserable and during the night Beverly started bleeding from one side of her face. Elaine had to take her back to the doctor the next morning to be drained. Ultimately, her surgery turned out all right, but the whole ordeal and the recovery experience was much more difficult than both she and her sister had expected, and Elaine never did go back to have her face done after that.

Operating times for surgery

Type of surgery	Average time for operation
Facelift with Eyelids	4–6 hours
Upper or Lower Eyelids	1–2 hours
Upper and Lower Eyelids	2–3 hours
Browlift-Open or Endoscopic	1–2 hours
Facelift	2–3 hours
Neck Liposuction	Less than 1 hour

Lift attendants

Women having cosmetic surgery deserve to be smothered with acts of kindness, chicken soup and loads of TLC. And I don't mean the kind you expect from your beau on your anniversary. I mean the kind that you can only get from your mother or granny when you ran a fever and had to stay at home from school. After the lift is the time you want to be treated like a princess and nothing less will do. Whenever possible, send your husband or paramour (or both) out of town or plan surgery around prolonged business trips. Even if they want desperately to take care of you, you're better off in the hands of a professional nurse who actually knows her way around dressings and wounds. No one looks glamorous after an interlude with a scalpel, and the harsh realities of surgery take some of the mystery out of how you stay looking so great. When my friend saw my battered neck after liposuction, he said that I looked like I had been attacked by Jack the Ripper. Now, if you are having your breasts trimmed or raised, you might think to involve your partner in the process, since he thinks he has a stake in their ownership already. Your fleshy face tissues are another story entirely and they are yours to do what you like with.

Rule number one: Don't go through surgery alone.

Rule number two: Tell as few people as possible.

They don't hand out purple hearts for women who nurse themselves after a facelift. GP Dr Horsewood-Lee emphasizes the importance of post-operative domestic arrangements. 'You can expect to look awful but are usually beginning to feel great fairly quickly. Your family must be prepared for it, or if you prefer to be totally clandestine, book yourself into a great halfway house hotel, rather than into a regular hotel where they won't be able to cope with your needs.' You need a support system, but not so much of a support system that could be called a crowd. Small children can be traumatized by seeing mummy bruised, swollen and looking like a monster, so warn them or, better still, send them off to Granny's for a week. If you hated having visitors and well-wishers the morning after your Caesarean, après your facelift is infinitely worse.

Common medications used in cosmetic surgery

Painkillers   Paracetamol, paracetamol with codeine, Co-Codamol
                    (Panadol Ultra, Paracodol, Paramol).
Antibiotics   Cephalexin (Ceporex, Keflex).
Anti-virals   Famcyclovir (Valtrex, Famvir).

The last thing you want to worry about after surgery is where to get eye pads and sterile swabs. If you live alone or don't want to impose on family or friends, private nursing attendants can be arranged by the hospital or your surgeon's office to care for you at home. It makes a big difference to have someone by your side to reassure you and keep you comfortable. The cost is about £15–20 per hour, which translates to about £180–240 per 12-hour shift. Some women may be temperamentally unsuited to having someone wait on them hand and foot, but for the first 24-hour period you won't regret it. According to Data Hartman, a former nursing administrator who is now a medical management consultant, the nurse–patient relationship is a delicate one. 'Patients are not aware of what surgery entails and the side effects of anaesthetics, scars and the healing process. They often don't realize they go into the hospital feeling right as rain and can't predict how they will feel after surgery. The majority of patients are sent home the day of surgery or the day after with no support at all.' This view of the patient–nurse relationship works both ways, however. 'The ideal patient is one who is relaxed, well informed and coachable,' says cosmetic surgery nurse Barbara Rhea. 'Serenity is key.' So, while you don't exactly have to sweet-talk your nurse, you should try not to treat her like the previous queen was beheaded and you've suddenly taken over the throne.

Nursing station
Recovery tips from the pros
According to nurses Barbara Rhea, RN, and Frances McGibbon, RN, NP, these are the key elements of making your recovery swift and efficient:

- Keep lips moist with an emollient sheer gloss applied with a wand applicator.
- When you are able to wash your hair, use gentle shampoo or baby shampoo and a spray-on detangler. Finger-comb only and avoid brushing and blow-drying at first.
- For your first visit to the clinic for suture removal, don't bother with makeup, moisturizer or sunscreen. Just leave your face bare.
- Sleep is a great healer. It allows your body to repair cells.
- Minimize your talking and chewing so facial muscles can rest.
- Be good to your skin. The trauma of surgery leaves skin feeling dry, itchy and sensitive and craving moisture.
- Don't wait until you are in excruciating pain to wave the white flag. Tell your carer as soon as discomfort sets in.
- Keep your mobile away from swollen ears after facial surgery. Rub it down with alcohol before use – or preferably switch to a speakerphone.

After surgery is a time to think 'convenience', except of course if you live in England. What makes Great Britain so great are London's brilliant black cabs that are surgically clean with an abundance of headroom, working parts and drivers who know how to get you home at the speed of light through back alleys. However, it is also the land of chemists and health shops that usually aren't open late at night or during the weekend. For this reason, you must plan ahead. Make sure your prescriptions are collected well in advance.

Don't overdose on vitamins either. Around 1000mg of Vitamin C is plenty; the preferred way to get it is from a real food source instead of a capsule. Imedeen, the Danish vitamin and mineral tablet from the sea, is a favourite supplement for pre- and post-facial surgery, as it has been specially developed to keep skin healthy and strong.

The best company after a lift might just be an endless supply of videos and a fridge stocked full of nutritious goodies.

Home, sweet home

You will be able to walk slowly out of the hospital or clinic to a waiting car with some assistance. That would be 'walk', as in not skipping, trotting or taking a taxi to the airport for a flight. This is no time to fuss about in your Jimmy Choos or Manolo Blahniks, either. Once safely at home, proceed without delay to the room where you will be staying for most of the next 24–72 hours. It is best to rest in a room with a loo on the same floor to avoid having to walk up and down stairs. Change into a comfortable, loose-fitting nightgown, robe or tracksuit with necklines that do not have to be pulled over your head, and settle in to rest. Slip on skid-free socks if you've got bare wood floors and stairs. Use your old bed linens, as there is likely to be soiling and staining of your sheets.

Set up an extra few fluffy pillows in the bed for added comfort and use waterproof pillow protectors to avoid soiling. Rest at home with moderate activity as tolerated for 48 hours, which translates to no physical exertion, driving, bending, carrying, lifting, exercise or sexual activity of any kind for a minimum of 10 days. Keep water at your bedside to swallow pills. You will be instructed on how to keep your suture lines clean and your dressings intact, if you have any.

An early, consistent use of ice packs over strategic areas for the first 24–48 hours can really cut down on swelling, bruising and tenderness. Never put ice packs directly on your skin, but wrap them first in a soft flannel or towel. Don't squander valuable brain cells agonizing over whether to use frozen petit pois or sweetcorn kernels, gel masks or ice chips. The goal is simply to apply cold to the area and expensive contraptions are not required. The 'no frills' method of dipping a flannel or gauze square into a bowl of iced water and then squeezing it out before applying it to the affected area works just as well.

Watch out for signs of infection near the incisions, such as increased swelling, redness, bleeding or other discharge. If you experience any unusual symptoms, report them to your doctor right away. Expect some bruising in the area of the incisions in front of the ears, on the neck and around the eyelids. There will be the most bruising where the most tension is, usually around the ears, and it may get worse over the first 48–72 hours. Avoid getting up from a sitting position or out of bed too quickly.

You may feel lightheaded for a few days after surgery. Keep one hand to steady yourself at all times or ask for help. You'll be asked to check that your bowels are functioning normally, as constipation is common. Your doctor may allow you to take a stool softener to avoid straining, which can cause additional swelling and pressure on suture lines. Keep dressings dry and do not shower or bathe until your doctor allows it, which is hopefully in a day or two. You may need some help bathing. Hold on to something in the bathroom to steady yourself and avoid using too hot or too cold water; lukewarm or tepid is best. You will be instructed to avoid smoking, alcohol, Vitamin E, aspirin or non-steroidal anti-inflammatory drugs (NSAIDs) for 2 weeks after surgery. Keep smokers at bay as well during your healing process.

You will not look like yourself immediately following a lift, but this is only a temporary condition. There is sometimes a period of emotional depression at the time when you look your worst, about 72 hours or so after the operation. Your hormone levels change after surgery, and you may start to feel sad or scared that you will not look like yourself again. Susan Harvey, President of Home Recovery Cosmetic Surgery Comfort Catalog, who developed a collection of kits for pre- and post-surgery after she had a little work done herself, says, 'Don't assume the success of your surgery is only up to your surgeon. The key is in the planning.'

Good food

- No dairy products – stay away from cream and cheeses, etc.
  Avoid spicy or greasy foods – no curries or Tandoori.
- Stick to a soft diet of clear broths, puddings and fruit smoothies –
  toddler foods like apple purée, scrambled eggs, mashed potato, etc.
- A bed tray is helpful for eating meals in bed.
- Drink lots of water, fruit juice, herbal caffeine-free teas or sports drinks.
- Avoid salt, garlic and preservatives.
- Sip liquids through a straw if you have had laser around the mouth.
  After 3 days, you can start on pasta and fish.

the importance of not being earnest
– tried and true excuses to tell the neighbours

The British tradition of maintaining personal privacy at all costs is a double-edged sword when it comes to cosmetic surgery. It is that very longstanding cultural idiosyncrasy that is responsible for creating the current climate of secrecy surrounding lifts. Deciding whether to go public about a lift or other surgery is a big decision. Although you may think that you getting lifted is a matter of the utmost importance to the Commonwealth, I assure you it is not. The act of confiding in even one lifelong friend you hold near and dear about your facelift is, in essence, telling the world. Once your secret is out, it is no longer safe. Don't be surprised to read about it in the dailies by the week's end. The possibilities are doom-laden.

After your lift, you will feel like you are living in a fishbowl, but if you plan as though Hyacinth Bucket is your next-door neighbour, you will be prepared for all eventualities. As such, you may bolt the doors and windows and lock yourself in during the day and only venture out at night, except if there's a full moon. Nearby acquaintances should only be informed about your surgery on a need-to-know basis.

In some respects, coming clean and telling all and sundry about your lift gives you the advantage of having the upper hand. You are able to control to a certain extent what is said about your lift. Only then (as most women do) do you have the option of downsizing a full facelift to 'just a little work around the eyes'. Lying about cosmetic surgery is like lying about your biological age by a decade or so. If you deny everything, they will assume it's much worse than it really is. If you leave people to speculate, a little collagen can turn into snide backhanded comments like, 'No wonder Marge looks so good. She's had a lot of work done you know…' The childhood game of Chinese whispers springs to mind, where the original message becomes distorted and exaggerated down the line until it is rendered virtually indistinguishable to its final recipient.

No excuses

It's up to you whether you want every man and his wife to know about your cosmetic surgery. Here you can weigh up the options about what you tell people:

The Truth v.	The Fib
Face- and necklift	A mini tuck
Facelift	Fat injections
Upper and lower eyelids	Fat bag removed
Lower eyelids	Laser peel
Neck liposuction	Personal trainer
Browlift	BOTOX

In my experience, the best way to manage the damage control is to scale it back. Be consistent. Never assume that your schoolmate Alice rarely talks to your aunt Suzanne, so they won't exchange notes. With your luck, there will be an exhibit at the Tate Modern of Post-

Impressionist water lilies that neither will want to miss and they'll bump into each other the very weekend you've told only one of them about having your eyes done. 'Have you seen Anne?', 'No, she's resting after her operation', 'What operation?', 'Oh, didn't she tell you about her eyes?', 'What happened to her eyes?', blah, blah, blah... Women are very funny about being each other's confidante. Not telling a supposed 'best friend' about having your eyes done is paramount to having an affair; if word gets out and you haven't told, your old best friend may feel betrayed.

When to have it done

The other hard part about having cosmetic surgery is the scheduling of it. Choosing when to get lifted requires careful and diligent planning. There are numerous factors to consider, not necessarily in this order: social commitments, family events, workload, the children's school terms, holidays, when your period is due and so forth. You also need to work round your surgeon's schedule. Some of the top surgeons are booked for 6 months to a year in advance, and picking a mutually convenient date to do your face can end up giving you wrinkles. Queue-jumping is not a simple matter either, unless you are willing to abandon all pride and resort to begging and pleading.

A host of seasonal issues will also prevail. Winter remains the top season for chemical peels and lasers, and spring and winter are most popular for facelift and eye procedures. No matter how carefully you plan, something will always come up to make the 'perfect' surgery date next to impossible. It's like getting pregnant; there is never a 'perfect' time. You'll have to miss out on something: your tennis season, a golf tournament, a ski trip to Cortina, your best friend's son's wedding, an unexpected christening, or the social event of the season. Stay away from toddlers and public transport because if you happen to catch the sniffles a couple of days before your surgery date, the anaesthetist might cancel you. If that's your only window of time, you may have to wait another year to have it done.

As with eating oysters, your best bet when it comes to scheduling your facelift surgery is to stick with months that have an 'R' in the name: January, February, March, April...

As Dr Horsewood-Lee says, 'The whole philosophy of cosmetic surgery runs completely counter to the huge complementary movement in the UK. Where dinner table talk from middle-class professionals is more likely to be about anti-ageing vitamins and growth hormones, these are the same people who are having their surgery secretly in January, definitely the boom month for quiet operations.'

Making your post-op debut

There is an unspoken law in cosmetic surgery: the woman who is planning to host a banquet for a visiting foreign dignitary 10 days after an eyelift will be the one in a thousand who will end up with a puffy purple spot under one eye that looks like her spurned lover took a swing at her. You must also make sure NEVER to schedule surgery right before your surgeon is going on a month's holiday in Cap Ferrat. Make sure he is around for at least one week, preferably two, so if you are having a problem, the man you handed over pots of money to is there to see you through it, rather than his senior registrar.

Another truism in cosmetic surgery is that if you follow your instructions to the letter and rest for the first 48–72 hours after surgery, your chances of healing faster skyrocket. The day after a complicated eyelid surgery, one of my Palm Beach clients invited me to join her at an antique auction at Sotheby's, so I threatened to tie her to the bedrail in her hotel suite. Another patient, a high-powered executive, tried to negotiate with me over what her surgeon really meant when he instructed her not to see her personal trainer for a month. I said he meant 4 weeks, 30 days, 2 fortnights. 'C'mon, my face isn't going to fall down is it?' After I assured her it would indeed, we settled on calling her doctor after 2 weeks to check. Listen to your doctor, nurse and carer. You're all on the same team (for real). This is one time that you should follow your mother's advice: keep quiet and be a good girl.

The healing process

Doctors have less control over how you heal than you might think. God is really at the helm when it comes to healing, but the obvious confusion between the two forces is understandable. Some people just heal better than others. Put away your magnifying mirrors, ladies, and bear down. The bruising resolves within 3–4 weeks, but the months following a facelift operation bring many changes. Although you can get on with your life within a reasonable amount of time, you will not be fully healed within a few weeks. Swelling, scar tissue formation, redness, tightness and discolorations are all part of the process and will follow their own course. The little lumps and bumps take months to soften up. At first, the neck will feel tight and stiff and your face will look as swollen as a pumpkin. As the swelling subsides, your nerves regenerate and you will start to feel tingling sensations. Ignore girlfriends who proclaim emphatically that they didn't have any bruising at all. Patients often forget the details of the lift experience. It's like childbirth; if we remembered how excruciating it was, no one would ever have a second child. Every lifted face has some degree of bruising. This ranges from a faint greenish discoloration to a deep red and purple haematoma. Scars that start out as red will fade to pink and eventually to finer lines over several months. But it won't happen overnight.

Surgically challenged skin needs a regime to nourish and protect it, coupled with a chemical-free sunblock, without overloading the skin and minus the perfumes, dyes or harsh additives. What you do to your facial skin pre- as well as post-lift, will help determine how quickly you sail through the healing. According to nurse Rikki Allen, 'A combination of glycolic peels, moisturizing facials and lymphatic massage will allow the skin to become more hydrated and elastic prior to surgery and therefore easier to operate on and prone to faster healing afterwards.'

Post-lift care – speedy healers
- SkinCeuticals Primacy C + E serum
- SkinCeuticals Primacy Phyto +
- Astara Conscious Skincare Microclusters Anti-Oxidant Infusers
- Jurlique Herbal Extract Recovery Gel
- BioMedic Clinical SkinCare Gentle Healing Ointment
- Karin Herzog Switzerland Vit-A-Kombi

The real deal on recovery

Before you start planning your diary events, read this section carefully so that you won't have to cancel over-optimistic appointments.

Back to work (BTW)

This is the earliest possible date when you can put on theatrical makeup, fix your hair and walk down the high street without children gawking at you. This is also the time when you are looking and feeling 'semi-normal' although surely not your best, and can pop into a sandwich shop for a coffee without scaring anyone away.

Mother of the bride (MOB)

This is a 'safe' date and considerably longer than BTW, when you can be reasonably certain that you will look 'well rested' and good enough to raise only a few suspicions among your dearest acquaintances, but long after the telltale signs are well concealed. It's fine for any major event such as your daughter's wedding, hosting a champagne brunch for the firm's managing director or going on safari in Kenya.

Upper eyelid tuck
Stitches out: 4–7 days
BTW: 7 days
MOB: 3 weeks

Lower eyelid fat bag removal
Stitches: none
BTW: 5 days
MOB: 2 weeks

Upper and lower eyelids
Stitches out: 4–7 days
BTW: 10 days
MOB: 3 weeks

Neck liposuction
Stitches: dissolvable
BTW: 4 days
MOB: 2 weeks

Browlift
Stitches and/or staples out: 10 days
BTW: 10 days
MOB: 4 weeks

Facelift
Stitches out: 10 days
Dressing off/drain out: 1–2 days
BTW: 10 days
MOB: 4–6 weeks

Laser resurfacing
Dressings removed: next day
BTW: 10 days
MOB: 4–6 weeks

If you are a smoker, have issues with authority figures, are prone to misbehaving when it comes to following instructions or if you are in the midst of high stress (i.e. embroiled in a nasty divorce, closing on a new flat or redecorating your drawing room), plan to add an extra few days to weeks to the above calculations. The better advice would be to postpone your surgery until you can map out a quieter time in your life to do it that will allow you to focus on taking care of yourself.

The bruise cycle

This is the typical life cycle of a bruise. This course varies from one face to another and one bruise to another, but takes 2–3 weeks in most people. Thinner skin, such as that around the eyelid area, bruises more than other areas of the face, as does the side or area that requires the most work.

1. Dark solid purple to mottled purple
2. Fading to bits of purple in green
3. Fading to green and yellow
4. Fading to yellow
5. Gone

the cover story

To get you through the initial healing phase, the next best investment you can make in your facelift (apart from a good plastic surgeon) is a good concealer. The real answer to the question 'how long will it take to heal?' is when you can go out without attracting attention, and by that I mean looking semi-normal when wearing camouflage. The better your camouflage, the sooner you can resume your daily routine.

Perfect tools

Use the thickest, densest cover-up you can find. Liquid and cream concealers usually won't work because they are not opaque enough. If the cream is too thick or too hard, first warm it up on your forehand. Skin texture changes after trauma to the skin so your normal concealer won't adhere in the same way on your post-lifted skin. Choose the shade that matches your skin tone or a slightly lighter shade. Do a swatch test on your jawline to see if it matches your skin. Practise applying your concealer near a window where there is indirect daylight to magnify flaws. Start with clean, dry skin. Coat an edge of a sponge with a generous amount of cover-up. Lightly pat (don't rub) the coated portion of the sponge on top and around the outside of the area to be disguised until you can no longer see the mark(s). Pat the outermost portion of the made-up area to blend the edges of the make-up so there is the illusion of no make-up at all. Try not to touch anywhere other than these lines of demarcation. A professional concealer brush will also help to place camouflage just where you want it.

The art of concealing flaws

1. Never put anything on an oozing wound before your doctor gives you clearance.
2. A sloppy application of concealer will draw more attention to your bruises.
3. Don't attempt to wear makeup before you REALLY must.
4. Use a good cleanser to remove every last drop of makeup.
5. Rubbing anything vigorously on your face will disturb the healing process.
6. Forget about covering up a deep purple bruise – you're wasting your time.
7. Buy concealer before the lift to have on hand when you need it.
8. Get professional help. Choose products where there is someone to guide you.

Blend your foundation face makeup gently around and slightly on top of the edges of the concealer. If your concealer is off-colour, gently pat the face makeup over it until the colour blends well with the rest of your face. Apply a translucent pressed or loose powder in a shade close to your skin-tone, or slightly lighter, to keep the make-up from mixing with the natural oils from your skin and melting. Avoid conscious and subconscious face-touching as this can wipe away your camouflage job. Take a very small amount of powder on the tip of a blush (or powder) brush and lightly (barely touching your skin) dust over the camouflaged area until the area is matt, or has the same sheen as the rest of your face. Keep a powder compact with you to touch up any shine over the course of the day.

According to makeup designer Stephen Glass, 'There is a balance as to how far one should go to throw people off the scent, depending on the degree of change to the face. Proper camouflage techniques are absolutely essential for confidence and feeling normal. Every woman needs a makeup update after surgery, but changes should be subtle, not extreme, for the wearer's sake as well as the onlooker's.'

Flawless
The best bets for covering up:
- Cover Care from Jane Iredale Mineral Cosmetics
- La Prairie Professional Cover Cream SPF15
- Bobbi Brown Essentials Professional Concealer
- Vincent Longo Cream Concealer
- Clinique Continuous Coverage
- Estée Lauder Maximum Cover SPF 15

You'll have to be clever to get around the hosts of unwelcome 'nosy parkers' you want to avoid. If you've been waiting for an occasion to break out the pashmina you got from Saint Nick last year in that questionable shade of green, now's your chance. Nothing hides a multitude of post-surgery signs as well. Another good cover-up after surgery is with a wide-brimmed hat that has a self-attached scarf to tie round your head. Clothing for protection from sun, rain, wind and cold is good, too. Sunglasses are a must-have, and not the sporty kind like Persol with the fine wire frames. You'll need the big, black, bold and bulky glasses with wide sides to conceal half your upper face, as favoured by Greta Garbo. If you're not sure if they are big enough, take this simple test: buy a standard size, rigid spectacles case. If your glasses fit into that case, they're way too small. Think goggles!

The unveiling – tips for throwing them off the trail
by face designer, Pablo Manzoni

You just took 10 years off your face, now do the same with your makeup. When you lift your face, you should lighten your makeup. Too many women have cosmetic surgery to enhance their looks and then go back to the same makeup they always used. There are two stages to the lift: 2 weeks later when you have to use heavy makeup to cover everything, and 2 months after, when the swelling has gone down. Once your face has settled in, it will be time to rethink your hair, makeup and wardrobe.

- Update your eyeglasses. Choose a frame slightly larger than what you have been wearing and tinted with lenses that go from darker to lighter from the top down. Dark circles under the eyes will look lighter by contrast.
- Avoid wearing earrings until your doctor expressly allows it. Start out with something small and light at first. If your lobes are still numb, use eyelash glue on the clips to keep your earrings on.
- Keep hair as long as possible around the ears before surgery to camouflage bruising. Have a stylist cut and reshape your hair 3 weeks after the lift to emphasize your newly rejuvinated jawline and neck. If you go short, leave some height at the top and wisps of hair around the ears and on the neck. Fringes, if needed, should be kept soft. Aim for a more upswept look all around.
- Cover your grey. You don't have to go lighter but a lifted face with grey roots showing is self-defeating.
- Take an inventory of your cosmetic collection and toss out anything over one year old or in a shade too dark or too glossy. Brighten up your makeup palette with only tones and textures that flatter. This is no time to experiment with fads and trends. Stick with safe, classic makeup that enhances your lifted face.
- Your new face needs new foundation. Choose one that is light-reflecting in a creamy, healthy shade for your skin type. The texture of your skin will be different, i.e. tighter and possibly oilier. Stick with oil-free formulas that are not too drying to avoid shine.
- A good eyebrow shaping is a must and they should not be too dark. Your eyes will need definition and should be lined as though they are framed to avoid looking naked. Stick to matt eyeshadows in neutral tones but add a touch of shimmer shadow to the browbone and the centre of the lid for warmth.

Case history

A week after my dear friend Nancie had a lift her mother-in-law had a massive coronary and passed away. Nancie, although never really fond of the old lady, thought she would go mad. 'This is her final plan to ruin me with the family,' she exclaimed, with her neckbands so tight she could barely get the words out. Desperate not to let her wicked sister-in-law spill the beans, I sent her a genius stylist to fix up her hair and face, lent her my treasured old Versace glasses from the early 80s that have been passed around from girlfriend to girlfriend over the years. We pulled out a cowl neck cashmere sweater, wrapped her head in an Hermes scarf so she looked like a grieving film star from the 1940s. No one suspected a thing at the funeral, in fact, she scored points with her husband's brothers who were genuinely touched at what they perceived as tears behind her dark glasses.

Jane Iredale
President of Iredale Mineral Cosmetics

- **Would you consider doing something radical like a lift or laser?**
  I've already done laser. I don't see going through life with something that makes you miserable if it can be improved.
- **What is your 'must-have' beauty treatment?**
  I was blessed with good English skin, but I need a very good moisturizer and I look for active ingredients. The 'anti-ageing' product I use every day is Cellex-C serum because I believe the research!
- **If you could go back in time, what would you do to keep wrinkle-free?**
  Avoid the sun! Thankfully, I grew up in Middlesex where we didn't see much of it and I stopped admitting to my real age when I was 21 so I'm not going to break a good habit.

once is not enough

As long as a woman can look ten years younger than her own daughter, she is perfectly satisfied

Oscar Wilde, *The Picture of Dorian Gray*

A common misconception of cosmetic surgery is that once you have a facelift, you'll have to keep having them. That depends on how you look at it. Having BOTOX first and then thinking about having a lift is not the same as taking paracetamol with codeine for a migraine one day and making a giant leap next to heroin. If you ask how long a facelift will last, the answer is forever. You will always look better for having had a lift at whatever stage you do it. As the face continually changes with age, the benefits of having a lift will ensure that you will look younger than your chronological age. There are those women among us for whom a facelift will be a one-off event, but I assure you they are becoming rarer. Even though you may be convinced that you are never going to do this again, my advice is to start saving your pennies for your second lift sooner rather than later. Think of it like your pension fund and consult your trusty banker. A wise investment locked away at today's rates will no doubt prosper and multiply sufficiently to counteract the staggering fee increase you can expect.

If you have your first lift at 45 or 50, you will easily have time for two more lifts in your lifetime. If you have one every decade or so, that would only bring you to retirement age. Short of bringing on the masking tape, rubber bands, thumb tacks and Super Glue to hold it all together, it is reasonable to assume that you will be up for at least considering another round somewhere down the line.

Famous last words

'I don't want to be pulled too tight.'
'I want to look natural.'
'I don't expect to look 25 again.'
'I don't want to look different.'
'I'm not telling anyone I'm having it done.'
'I never thought I'd be doing this.'
'I've always looked young for my age.'
'I'm only going to do this once.'

staying gorgeous - the art of maintenance

The fine art of maintenance is a lifestyle approach to prolonging the results of a lift for as long as possible through sensible living, advanced skincare and occasional beauty shots and skin treatments. Although there is a faction of women who believe that 'para' surgical treatments are akin to something in the realm of 'para' normal, the rest of us are already hooked. You owe it to yourself and your bank account to protect your investment from the perils of the environment, sun, wind, cold and those evil free radicals. Free radicals may sound like a throwback to the era of macramé, tie-dye and bell-bottoms, but their effects are far more devastating than merely a low point in the annals of fashion. They are destructive little molecules that cause photo-ageing, damage DNA and RNA, contribute to skin cancer and can ruin your hard-earned lift. The free radical problem has worsened in recent years due to pollution, pesticides, radiation, smoking and the general wearing down of the ozone layer. The best defence you've got is an all-out campaign to hide from them, and adopt therapies that go on a search and destroy mission to neutralize them.

Making it last

Factors that affect how long your lift will last:
- Your age at the time of the lift.
- The condition of your skin.
- Genetics.
- Emotional state.
- Diet and nutrition.
- Surgical technique used.
- Sun exposure.
- Smoking.
- Excessive drinking.

Lift tracking

You always look great for the first year after a lift, but keep records of the little flaws that will appear at intervals. As the swelling goes down after your lift, note the flaws every 3 months, 6 months and 12 months.

The first year after your lift, the wrinkles will start to reappear. Note when and where they appear every 2 years, 3 years, 4 years and 5 years.

Second time around

Helen Bransford, the 50-something author of *Welcome To Your Facelift*, opens up about life after the lift…

● **After your facelift did you get hooked on cosmetic surgery?**

For me, no way. I revelled in the result of my 'face retrieval', which seems more apt than 'lift'. Since then, the science that swirls around beauty has exploded from matchstick to raging forest fires and the geography of my own life has shifted. I understand the temptation to re-open Pandora's box, but it's frighteningly easy to lose perspective and have a new procedure every 18 months. I long to rest on the laurels of my surgeon (Mr Dan Baker in New York), and take only tiny steps as new atrocities are revealed.

My strategy is to avoid the operating room via good health and rigorous maintenance. The nasty little secret is that appearance and self-esteem are umbilically linked in all of us. Even my mother insisted packaging was half the battle.

● **What is your advice for making the lift last?**

The newsflash is that basic grooming has quietly evolved into high-tech art form that laces in and out of the medical arena. Pharmaceutical-grade skincare products, an occasional foray into BOTOX, a peel to contain sun damage, clean healthy teeth, an occasional micro-dermabrasion, a stitch to target the errant sag, maybe an injectable filler to plump out canyons, and a watchful eye on the progress of lasers.

● **If you could turn the clock back, what anti-wrinkle strategy would you follow?**

In a word, common sense. For 30 years I tortured and baked the creamy skin I was born with in an effort to force a tan and look as smart as everyone else. The damage is still rising to the surface (karma in action, I presume) and the lines around my eyes are in need of some serious discipline. Today I live by own cobbled rules: No dawdling in the sun (talk to someone else about Vitamin D absorption), no basking in second-hand smoke (or first- or third-hand either), concentrating on living foods, seizing every chance to sneak in some exercise and rigorously avoiding the following demons: sleep deprivation, heavy flirting with drugs or booze, and extreme contortion of my face to make babies laugh (or cry). The most tedious words my mother uttered, I now embrace as my credo: moderation in all things. Burning the candle at one end is more than enough.

trigger events

Your first facelift may have been triggered by the usual things like weddings, divorces, job changes, retirement or an expected inheritance from a great-aunt. Your second facelift is a different sort of occurrence. It is a little like marriage number two; you worried more with the first one but now you feel like you know what you're doing and are less nervous.

Your comfort level is higher this time as you already know what to expect. The exception would be if your previous foray into cosmetic surgery had been a disaster, which will make you more apprehensive the second time round because of the memories it will dredge up. Fortunately, the latter scenario is far rarer. After your first lift, you are no longer a novice. You are a seasoned and experienced patient and your standards are far greater.

The results of facial rejuvenation surgery on younger patients are less dramatic because there is less to be done. Similarly, the results of secondary facelifts and eyelid procedures are also more subtle. After the first facelift, future facial tightening procedures will require a more moderate approach. The big work will have already been done on the deeper layers, and so just the skin and more superficial tissues are tweaked down the road.

Secondary procedures are far more refined. You can't expect to turn the clock back 10 years every time you have a lift. Do the maths. That would mean that if you started at 45, by your third lift you would look around middle-school age. The degree of change you will get from a second facelift is universally more subtle than the original one, and if there is a third, it will be even more so.

Finesse is the main ingredient to successful subsequent facial cosmetic surgeries. Overdoing it after the tissues have already been worked on is far more risky. Trifling alterations, such as taking in a seam here and making a dart there, should suffice. According to Mr Brian Coghlan, 'Usually women who are on their second or third facelift need only minor revisions or they can end up with a wind-swept look. We try to go to a different level, deeper or more superficial, combined with fat transfers around the mid-face. Positioning of the scars becomes an issue also, and we try to use the existing scar or make the incision on the lower border of the hairline.' The good news is that after the first lift, the second and third should be a breeze. At the staggering rate that the world of cosmetic surgery appears to be changing, by the time you are ready for the next round, you can expect significant improvements in terms of healing times, anaesthetics and technology, as well as more natural and better-quality results. The downside is that you will be older, and so will your tissues.

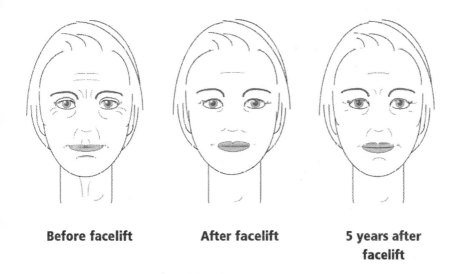

Before facelift   **After facelift**   **5 years after facelift**

There are three types of cosmetic procedures: temporary, semi-permanent and permanent, with some variables. For example, an open forehead lift (where hair-bearing skin is removed) is usually done only once in a lifetime, whereas a lower facelift may be done every 5–10 years.

Longevity of a facial procedure

- TEMPORARY
  Upper eyelids – fat only
  Lower eyelids – fat only
  Neck liposuction
  Endoscopic facelift
  Endoscopic browlift
  Laser resurfacing
- SEMI-PERMANENT
  Upper eyelids – fat/skin
  Lower eyelids – skin/muscle/fat
  Modified facelift (upper, lower)
  Face- & necklift
- PERMANENT
  Open browlift

preparing for round two

The next big dilemma is choosing the surgeon for your second lift. Although there is less to do in a secondary facial rejuvenation procedure, that does not necessarily mean that it is foolproof. In my mind, doing less and doing it well, often requires greater skill. I might not, for example, routinely recommend a junior surgeon straight out of training for a secondary face or necklift. There is a learning curve to managing the fine-tuning that comes with experience in doing both primary (the first time) and subsequent lifts. If you had a positive experience and were happy with your result the first time, nothing would delight your surgeon more than having you consult him again, unless of course you made a great pest of yourself and he has put a big black 'X' next to your name. In most cases, a reputable surgeon takes great pride in maintaining relationships with patients and would be honoured to have the opportunity to work on you again. By the same token, assuming some time has passed between lifts, he may also be senile, retired, struck off or deceased.

Just as techniques go out of fashion and newer ones replace them, one of the great injustices in cosmetic surgery is that the surgeon who did your face 10 years ago may no longer be on the 'A' list now, having less to do with his skills and expertise and more to do with his PR.

Case history

Maureen O'Shaunessy, 57, had a full facelift and her lower eyelids done by the now retired London plastic surgeon Mr Freddie Nicolle when she was just 46. She told absolutely no one about it, not even her husband who was in Dubai at the time or her daughter at school. Due to an ideal combination of Mr Nicolle's considerable skill and her fine-quality skin, she healed brilliantly and her scars are well concealed. To this day, they haven't a clue that she did anything at all to her face, and she looks younger than most of their friends who are her contemporaries. Only recently, 11 years after her original surgery, she is bothered by loose skin on her upper eyelids, fat bags in the corners, and the re-emergence of her jowls. Upon consulting with two prominent London plastic surgeons, Maureen was told she would be a good candidate to have a strip of excess skin and some fat removed from her upper eyelids (which had never been done before), as well as a lower facelift to tighten her neck and some laser resurfacing with Erbium:YAG for the fine lines around her eyelids and mouth. All in all, if she amortized the money she spent at age 46 out over eleven years, her early facelift proved to be a better investment than krugerrands.

One can plainly see that the better you take care of your lifted face and neck, the longer it will last. There are, however, some possible exceptions that can contribute to shortening its longevity. The types of faces on which even the best of lifts will not last well tend to be the ones that need the most attention to begin with. For example, the face of Arabella Churchill, who looks rather like her famous grandfather with breasts, was lifted live on the Internet on Celebritydoctor.com. A lifetime of tobacco indulgences and nipping at the cooking sherry surely got the better of her and, as such, she would not have been considered the ideal candidate for cosmetic surgery. A thick neck, square jaw and slack skin do not enhance your chances for having a brilliant lift. A surgeon will have far better odds at scoring a home run on a face like Julie Christie's or Elizabeth Taylor's. Great bones and skin are second only to a great surgeon.

Surgical challenges

The following are the factors that will make it more challenging to achieve a good facelift result:

- Fat face
- Thick neck
- Gaunt face
- Neck bands
- Thin skin
- Weak chin
- Long face

moderation in all things – just say no

Is not plastic surgery an art and the plastic surgeon an artist? The plastic surgeon works with living flesh as his clay, and his work of art is the attempted achievement of normalcy in appearance and function.

Jerome Pierce Webster, Chief of Plastic Surgery, Columbia College of Physicians and Surgeons

What facial rejuvenation surgery cannot do is turn Cruella de Ville into Cinderella. If a homely woman has a facelift, she will look younger, but she will still be homely. No facelift will transform her into Cindy Crawford. If that is what you were hoping for, you are setting yourself up to be disappointed. 'It is a mistake to try to choose the shape or style of a "new" feature. A surgeon can improve on your current looks, but cannot turn you into something or someone different. For example, a facelift will not change the shape of your face,' says Dr John Celin, and 'eyelid surgery cannot slant your eyes, nor should it'.

Case study

Jenny Taylor, 46, was considering having a lift. She settled on one for doing her eyelids, face and neck and an endoscopic browlift. She also saw a TV documentary about lip enhancement and thought she'd have her upper lip made fuller, too. Jenny was also toying with having some refinements to her nose. When she called the surgeon's office to ask about it, she was told to see the surgeon for a third consultation about the lips and nose. The result was that the surgeon talked her into leaving her nose alone and putting some of her own fat into her lips only. He felt she was doing too many things at the same time, and would look dramatically different. If she still wanted her nose done at a later date, that was fine. Jenny agreed and still has her old nose and is quite glad she does.

It is tempting to do a few procedures at once or close together, but it may not be as glamorous as it seems at first glance. Once you've healed up, you might not be as willing to dive right into the next procedure within a few months or even years. Minor alterations and maintenance therapies are not as much of an ordeal, but every time you alter one facial feature, your face will invariably appear differently to you. Good cosmetic surgery is practically invisible. You don't notice it. Bad cosmetic surgery is painfully obvious to all. You have to be able to identify what properly performed cosmetic surgery looks like in order to recognize the difference. According to Dr Bernard Cornette de Saint Cyr, 'A good result from a facelift is a good shape, good volume, good scars, good lobes and a good tragus.' The goal of modern plastic surgery is to enhance without distorting the natural contours of the face and its anatomical structures. It should not draw attention to itself; it should draw attention to you. Excellence in cosmetic surgery is an understanding of what ageing has done to change the face, achieving a harmonious change while maintaining the essence of beauty and without causing any undesirable side effects of surgery. As Dev Basra, FRCS says, 'I always believe in simplicity. With a variable of one, the number of things that can go wrong is none. With a variable of ten, the number of things that can go wrong is one thousand and twenty three.'

when enough is too much

...My girlfriend went back to her plastic surgeon. He told her, 'Sweetheart, you have nothing left to lift. If I do more, you're going to look worse.' Worse maybe, but younger...

From a Tracey Ullman sketch

Cosmetic surgery has an effect similar to certain mood enhancing drugs. It can seduce you like a swarthy stranger with a French accent and a wicked smile. Diving head first into addiction is always a lingering danger. There are inherent risks in becoming a 'cosmetic surgery junkie'. Women go to great lengths to achieve physical perfection but cosmetic surgery should not be looked upon as a fashion statement, fad or craze similar to ayurvedic spas or kickboxing. The business of beauty and beautification has a tendency to stimulate a wave of narcissism in its zeal to stamp out the stigma of ageing. But it all has to be kept in perspective. There is a fine line between self-improvement and self-obsession. Too much of a good thing can be a disaster; just witness some of Hollywood's most famous overdone faces that have been pulled, stretched, filled and sanded to the max.

The other side of the coin is that having multiple procedures is not quite as radical as it sounds. A woman who began with BOTOX and had her eyes done at 40, a lower facelift at 45 and at 50 is contemplating an upper face and browlift, is not an 'addict'. Addiction is when you are driven by forces greater than your own judgment to continuously tinker around with parts of your face to make yourself look different, better or prettier, when your features are reasonably fine as they are. There are two basic categories of cosmetic surgical procedures: surgery for ageing, and surgery for change.

Surgery that is undertaken to reverse the signs of ageing, for example, eyelid surgery, face- and necklifts and browlifts, is very different to the procedures that are intended to make you look different. Although it is just as common to become obsessed with reversing every line and wrinkle as they turn up, in my experience, surgery undertaken to change your look is infinitely more radical. When you keep transforming yourself, you lose a sense of your identity, of who you really are as an individual.

Surgery for change

Typically, cosmetic surgery to change how nature made you, rather than surgery to enhance and preserve what you inherited, includes:
- Nasal refinements
- Cheek augmentation
- Lip augmentation
- Lip lift
- Chin and jaw implants
- Pinning ears back

There is a huge rift between glamour and glitter. The overriding theme among cosmetic surgery junkies is that they all look like they have had surgery, and they all look strikingly similar. The character in their faces has been erased, their noses have been bobbed into oblivion, and they cannot wince, smile coyly or express hyper emotions. Women who have no sense of self can be sold, talked into or led to do anything.

The media frenzy that developed around one famous ex-wife of an international art dealer who 'nipped and tucked' herself to the point of no return, caused many questions to be raised about the ethics of cosmetic surgery. The real 'freaks' are not representative in any way of the typical women who undergo cosmetic procedures. Becoming unrecognizable is usually the result of multiple, aggressive procedures via surgery, injections, implantation, and to the skin itself, performed frequently over a long period of time – and often by several surgeons on numerous continents.

The skin is a living organ that can only withstand so much assault before it begins to take on an unnatural or waxy appearance. It should be noted that this look is often the patient's choice and is not necessarily what the surgeon recommends. There are women who simply insist on having a little 'tuck' here or there if they so much as see a wrinkle daring to form. The sad reality is that if one surgeon refuses to do the procedure, they will keep going until they find one willing to operate. If two or more surgeons tell you not to do it, go home and put it on the shelf for a spell. There will always be someone in Harley Street or elsewhere foolish or greedy enough to operate, even if it should not be done for medical, ethical and moral reasons. To those doctors, your sagging jowls represent a Brioni camelhair overcoat or a vintage platinum Patek Philippe, and they will not let it slip through their fingers without putting up a fight.

A good measure of reason is to listen to your friends. If they start suggesting that you're going over the top, perhaps it's time to give it a rest. Women are usually seeking the most 'bang for the buck' but often don't know what that is or where to draw the line on their own. Christina Carlino suggests, 'My biggest rule is one thing at a time. I cannot and will not embrace the idea of the total re-do. Choosing to alter your appearance should come from a healthy rather than an insecure place.'

Along with the growing list of syndromes of the psyche is BDD, or Body Dysmorphic Disorder. This refers to a culture of surgery groupies who will go to great lengths to change their looks. Women who are particularly vulnerable may easily fall into the trap of trying to re-make themselves via the scalpel. They have a distorted body image that leads to a host of compulsive, impulsive and anxiety problems including low self-esteem, eating disorders, depression, violence and suicide. In the BDD afflicted, a seemingly minor facial flaw becomes magnified so it is perceived as a very major and hideous deformity. They are often very secretive and may hide their neuroses from their plastic surgeon until afterwards. According to Dr David Veale of The Priory Hospital, an expert in BDD, 'Sufferers may demand perfection and an impossible ideal. There is a big disparity between what they believe they should ideally look like and how they see themselves. Many have repeatedly sought treatment with cosmetic surgeons with little satisfaction before finally accepting psychiatric help.' It's a slippery slope from experimenting to all out self-destruction.

The bottom line is that a new face does not guarantee a new life.

Liz Earle of Naturally Active, a natural skincare range

- **What is your regimen for de-ageing?**

  There is nothing wrong with growing old or looking older, but there is also no harm in looking your best, too! I am not a fan of 'miracle' creams that claim to stop ageing, but I do advocate that a little time and care will reap great results. Look after your skin regularly and don't just focus on your skincare routine: hand-in-hand with skincare is sleep – get plenty and not just 'enough'. Cleansing, toning and nourishing are the key regular skincare tenets, but I also swear by treating skin to a little frequent TLC, too.

- **Firming creams and toning exercise are not the only answer: what are your thoughts on facelifts and beauty shots?**

  Cosmetic surgery is invasive and so carries risks, so quite a bit of time needs to be spent considering the pros and cons before proceeding. Analyze the reasons why you want the surgery and think twice before a semi-permanent procedure. I think we need to be less 'hung up' about ageing – it's a positive thing: laughter lines simply mean we spend a lot of time smiling!

Fatal attraction

If your answer is number 4 to more than 3 of the following questions, skip the knife and log on to Prozac.com...

Which of these have you done in the past 2 years?

1. Followed a string of fad diets
2. Had CACI, CLEO and semi-permanent makeup
3. Had a tanning bed course and some self-tanning
4. Most or all of the above

Are you vacillating about having...?

1. Collagen Instant Therapy for your wrinkles
2. Your eyes and chin done now or later
3. Cheek implants and your nose shortened when you have your facelift and browlift
4. A total facial rejuvenation at the same time as your breast implants and liposuction

Do you want to cry because you hate the way you look in the mirror?

1. Never
2. Once in a while
3. Often
4. Always

Do you feel that everyone is prettier than you are?

1. Never
2. Once in a while
3. Often
4. Always

Do you feel so self-conscious about your looks that it is hard to enjoy being with people?

1. Never
2. Once in a while
3. Often
4. Always

9

in God we trust, but choose your doctor wisely

In a good surgeon, a hawk's eye, a lion's heart and a lady's hand.

Leonard Wright

Doctors fall into that vast category of professionals such as solicitors and barristers whose elevated stature is a matter of rank rather than explicit competence. In the UK, professional advice is quite highly regarded and generally deferred to. Placing your fate in someone else's hands alleviates the onerous burden of making the decision yourself. If you allow another person to choose for you, there is always someone to blame if things go wrong. Ultimately, the decision of selecting a cosmetic surgeon for your face is yours and yours alone. No one can really make the choice for you, nor should they.

Finding out who the good ones are is no small feat. You can't just go up to a woman in a shop or on the high street and say, 'Who did your face?'. Not only would it be an inexcusable invasion of privacy, but when it's good, there are few clues to help you sort out the lifted faces from all the others. If you are up for the challenge, you will need to muster the investigative skills of Deputy Chief Inspector Frost as well as the tenacity of Hetty Wainthrop.

Case history

Sandy Polk attended a holiday cocktail party and she spied an old friend, a fashion model who was around her vintage (the middle 60s). It was an intimate gathering, and their children had attended school together, so Sandy felt comfortable taking her friend aside and asking her with all deference, 'You look more beautiful every time I see you. I'm thinking about having a facelift and I'm so afraid. May I ask you, who do you use?' The woman was aghast. 'You dreadful woman,' she said, 'how dare you ask me such a personal question. My face is no one's business but my own,' and she marched to the other side of the room.

the best doctor

If you have even been tinkering with the idea of having some cosmetic work done, you have probably been collecting names of doctors from friends, other physicians, hairstylists and clippings from magazines and newspapers, and every source has its own favourites. Although recommendations from friends and acquaintances may seem helpful, they are sometimes more trouble than they are worth. 'You must go and see Mr Black, he's very good,' may not be enough of an endorsement to cause you to add Mr Black to your list unless you query a bit more: 'What makes him good? What is he good at? Who is he? Have you seen his work?, and so on. It isn't fair to judge a surgeon on the basis of one isolated recommendation, or condemnation either. Not every facelift is a grand slam on every patient, and you can never really know exactly what transpired from the before to the after. When the same name or clinic keeps coming up as one to avoid, it is wise to pay attention. The most important credential a doctor has is his professional reputation.

The real gift in cosmetic surgery is as much in the eyes as it is in the hands. If you know what beauty is but can't deliver it, it's just as tragic as knowing how to operate but being devoid of a sense of aesthetics. When I meet a surgeon, I look for those special qualities, such as a sense of creativity, raw talent, innovation and skills, coupled with some ray of light that tells me he actually cares about the patient. Not all surgeons are warm and fuzzy; in fact, some are downright nasty and arrogant. There is no substitute for skill and experience in a surgeon. You might overlook an awful bedside manner if his results are magical.

Fortunately, there are only a handful of really bad cosmetic surgeons, but sadly, just as few great ones. The bad ones should be relegated to females of a four-legged variety only. There are many good and very good surgeons that fall within the middle category. The real trick is discovering a diamond in the rough; the one who has the hands to be truly magical, but before he gets so famous that his head won't fit through the door. Some of the best surgeons I know make it a point to learn from the great ones. They watch them operate, perfect the technique and then tailor it to their own style. Some surgeons have it in their blood; when they enter the operating theatre, the instruments stand up and salute. If you want to know who has great hands, ask a nurse or an anaesthetist who watches them at work and has the tools as a basis for comparison.

In cosmetic surgery, there is rarely only one best doctor for any procedure. There are usually many who can execute a fine surgical plan. There is no magic formula to finding that one in a million. It should not be likened to seeking your one true soul mate with whom you are destined to spend the rest of your life. Some surgeons are generalists and can do most operations well. Others find their own niche – the one area they truly excel at and enjoy operating on.

Surgeons often get pigeon-holed into becoming known as 'the breast guy' or 'the best neck man', but skilled aesthetic surgeons can usually perform more than one operation like a master. Unlike many other fields of medicine, which treat diseases of mysterious origins, locating a good cosmetic surgeon is not as tricky if you determine what qualities are most important to you in a surgeon. Proper qualifications and training in an appropriate field is a given, but the rest can be very subjective. The 'BEST' doctor for your sister-in-law may not be the right one for you for a variety of reasons. According to Mr Norman Waterhouse, FRCS, 'To a patient who is looking for facial rejuvenation, the best recommendation is from other patients. It will make them feel more comfortable from the start.'

If you are planning to travel to another city or country, pick one where you have a close friend or relative to keep you company. You will be required to stay from one to two weeks after surgery before you can fly, and it gets lonely being on your own in a strange place. It may seem romantic to contemplate getting lifted across The Pond or the Channel, but if you consider the logistics, it may not always be practical. There is a certain degree of follow-up required after facial rejuvenation procedures that must be calculated into your decision. If you do have surgery in another city or country, unless your surgeon has a reciprocal professional relationship with a doctor in your geographical area, you will be left to fend for yourself. No plastic surgeon likes to take care of another doctor's surgical patients, especially if they are having a problem.

Choosing a surgeon

Rank these in order of importance to you from 1 to 10:
- Doctor congeniality (fab bedside manner)
- Accessibility (he'll call you back even on a Sunday if you're oozing)
- Warm and fuzzy staff (high TLC factor)
- Doc Hollywood (celebrity clientele)
- Booked (like getting a celebrity hairstylist to fit you in)

- Doc du jour (the flavour of the month)
- Designed with a capital 'D' waiting room (at the 'right' address)
- Natural look (leaves a little bit hanging)
- A bargain (he'll even put some fat in your lips for free)
- He'll do it in his office surgery (I won't have to go in to hospital)

doing your homework

Before scheduling a consultation with a surgeon, request brochures and develop a list of questions so you can discuss what is involved with a specific procedure. Force yourself to become Internet savvy or enlist the services of someone who can help you. Ask other specialists (not only your GP) for referrals. Make sure the surgeon is a reputable member of an organization of surgeons which specialize and that he has documented education, has completed a formalized training programme and has extensive experience in performing the procedures you are considering. Visit doctors' websites, and request a biog, practice leaflet and any other information sources about the procedures you are investigating. Get to know as much as you can about the surgeon before you make the appointment so you can save your valuable time and money.

Other factors to consider are fees, availability and your impression of how helpful and organized the staff is. Find out in advance about the range of fees so you can be prepared to stay within your budget. If you have a specific date in mind, some surgeons are booked way in advance but there is sometimes a waiting list for cancellations if you are willing to be flexible.

According to the General Medical Council (GMC), there are 36,199 doctors on the Specialist Register and some doctors are registered in more than one speciality. See your GP when you come down with the flu, but facelifts should be done by qualified cosmetic surgeons who have an eye for aesthetics. Make sure your surgeon is trained in both surgery and aesthetic surgery. 'FRCS', the acronym for Fellow of the Royal College of Surgeons (of England, Scotland

and Ireland), is only an indication that the surgeon has had basic surgical training. If the surgeon is trained in the UK, he should be listed in the GMC Specialist Register. If he is not UK-trained, then the same rules will apply in his own country of origin or where he did his training. If he is American for example, he should be 'board certified' in his speciality. Although just completing specialist training in plastic surgery or passing an exam is NOT a guarantee of excellence in aesthetic surgery, it is a place to start your search.

According to Geoff Benn of Nuffield Hospitals, 'Clinical governance will prohibit consultants from doing surgery outside their training because they must prove that they have substantial experience. At leading private hospitals like Nuffield, consultants have been checked out for proper qualifications and have substantial NHS practices.' At some clinics, however, surgeons can hang up a sign that says 'cosmetic surgeon' and start operating on patients without delay. A white coat is not always a solid indication of a real surgeon with sufficient training.

Once your first go at a list of surgeons is narrowed down, start scheduling your visits for an initial consultation. Most reputable surgeons will charge a consultation fee (roughly £75–150). The consultation visit can run half an hour to a full hour in some cases. Find out beforehand if you will be charged an additional fee for a second consultation. Most surgeons charge only the one consultation fee, even if you come back two or three times before your operation. It is reasonable to expect a surgeon to charge a fee for his time, and these fees can really add up if you are seeing several doctors. Be wary of 'free' consultations that are often a ruse to get you into the clinic. The old adage, 'you get what you pay for', rings true here. If you do your homework, you may be able to rule out some of the doctors on your list, based on what you find out even before you make your appointment.

The Surgical Career Path

These are the various stages in the career path of a cosmetic surgeon. It explains how a pink-faced 18-year-old becomes a consultant surgeon.

1. Medical School

Prerequisites	At least 3 good A-levels in appropriate subjects
Duration of training	5 years
Examination taken	MBBS, MBBCH
Qualification on completion	Provisional registration with the GMC

2. House Officer

Prerequisites	Provisional registration with the GMC
Duration in post	1 year
Examination	No examination
On completion	Full registration

3. Senior House Officer (SHO)

Prerequisites	Full registration with the GMC
Duration in post	2 years (minimum)
Examination	MRCS/AFRCS
On completion	MRCS/AFRCS

4. Specialist Registrar (SpR)

Prerequisites	MRCS/AFRCS
Duration	5 or 6 years, depending on specialization
Examination	Intercollegiate Examination (FRCS)
On completion	Certificate of Completion of Surgical Training

5. Consultant Surgeon

Pre-requisites	Must be in GMC's Specialist Register
Examination	Selected by Advisory Appointments Committee
Duration	Until retirement

(SOURCE: The Royal College of Surgeons of England)

the consultation visit

When you arrive, look around at the doctor's consulting rooms and at the other patients and the staff. Cosmetic surgeons will often operate on their secretaries and nurses. You can sometimes get a good idea of the type of work the surgeon does and the sort of clients he attracts by careful observation. At the very least, you will get a sense of the level of professionalism in his rooms and how he runs his medical practice.

One of the most common mistakes is to over-focus on one feature and miss something else that needs attention for an aesthetically pleasing effect. Try to avoid any preconceived notions about what you need to have fixed or improved: for example, fixating on your eyelids when it is your brows that need lifting; or having only your lower eyelids done, when your upper eyelids are falling fast. Get the doctor's opinion and suggestions instead of telling him what you think you need. Changing or rejuvenating one feature on the face will surely make the other features look different or older in comparison.

It is the universal practice of cosmetic surgery for a surgeon to hand you a mirror at the beginning of the consultation and ask you to show him what is bothering you: 'What can I do for you?', he will ask. If you're not sure, you shouldn't have made the appointment in the first place. That isn't to say that you MUST know exactly what you need on your own or be able to name the anatomical structure using scientific terminology. You should be able to explain as specifically as possible what you don't like about your face, what looks different or older than it used to and what, if anything, you want to change. It is your responsibility to let the surgeon know, not the other way around. Don't arrive at your consultation appointment with a blank slate.

Prepare a list of questions to bring with you to your consultation visit so you don't forget anything important to ask, and do take notes. You will forget most of what he tells you during the visit, and writing it all down will come in handy later on. Save the questions about fees, payment and scheduling for the doctor's secretary. This is not a time to be shy. Ask a lot of questions and ask to see pre- and post-op photographs of other patients he has operated on to get an idea of both his aesthetic skills and what results you can expect from the surgery. You need to know the basics of the procedure and how they apply directly to you: where the incisions are, what kind of anaesthetic, what hospital he operates in, how long the surgery is and so forth. If you get nervous during the consultation, you can forget something that may be important to ask. This is especially frustrating if you've waited half a year and another half a day in reception for your quarter of an hour appointment with a busy surgeon and he has one foot out of the door just as you remembered something you were dying to find out.

It is best to go alone to the first meeting. Your initial visit should be between the doctor and you, without any distractions. Leave well-meaning and curious girlfriends behind, and if your mate or spouse is not totally supportive, you would be wise to discourage him from accompanying you. If you absolutely have to have moral support, a daughter is usually the best choice. The first consultation visit is like a 'first date', to see if you and the doctor like each other and connect on some level. You also will want to find out if you feel comfortable with him and what he wants to do to you. It must be all about you, and you alone.

Case history

Susan Reynolds, 41, scheduled a consultation appointment with a very fashionable New York plastic surgeon. The next appointment available was 18 months hence, and she forgot all about it until a few days before when the office called to confirm. She quickly called her husband at work and told him that they had to go to New York. He cancelled his meetings, and she booked their airline tickets and a room at The Plaza to get there for her consultation. By now, she was already 42, and was thinking about having her neck done. The doctor greeted her, turned her neck from side to side, and said quite simply, 'You're not ready. Come back and see me again in two years,' and left the room. She didn't know whether to be happy or furious, so she went shopping instead and had a weekend in New York. Susan's was the most expensive five-minute consultation on record.

second opinions

There is no precise formula for choosing the right cosmetic surgeon. Ultimately, you have to use your own judgement and instincts. Never go with the first or only doctor you see; always get at least a second opinion, and preferably three or more, before you choose. It is not the British way to 'shop around', but with cosmetic surgery it is essential. Even if you may love the first doctor you see and feel comfortable with him, go and see at least one or two others for confirmation and comparison. After the third, you may still find you want to go with the first one you saw, but only after you see others are you really qualified to choose wisely. Finding the right cosmetic surgeon is a very personal journey. What appeals to one woman, may be totally inappropriate or offensive to another. Unless you feel comfortable with the surgeon and what he is recommending for you, wait and re-think it again, or go and see another surgeon, until it feels like a good fit. If it doesn't feel right, you should always keep going.

In the UK, there is great resistance to challenging the almighty Mr Doctor, whereas in the United States that went out along with Marcus Welby MD. Contrary to popular belief, questioning 'professional' judgement is not an act of treason. You do not have to feel that you have made a commitment to a surgeon after having had a consultation. There is no betrayal or cheating involved in getting a second opinion.

Once you have narrowed down your list to one or two surgeons, go back and see the frontrunner again. You should always see the surgeon who will be doing your surgery at least twice before the operation. The initial consultation and evaluation should be with the doctor and not a commissioned salesperson or the 21-year-old receptionist. The next visit is usually scheduled close to your operation date so you will have an opportunity to ask all the last-minute details you forgot to ask the first time or can't remember the answers you were given. This second meeting should leave you feeling content that you have made a wise choice. You may still have pre-lift jitters, but by this time you should have confidence in the surgeon.

Some of us spend more time shopping for a car than we do for a facelift – and there are no test drives when it comes to surgery. You owe it to yourself to approach cosmetic surgery as an empowered and educated consumer. If you shop for a camera, you don't just buy the first camera you see in the first camera shop you visit, and you don't shop for a Nikon at Russell & Bromley. Apply the same logic to the process of choosing a surgeon. Cosmetic surgery is not something you hear about today and pencil into your diary for tomorrow.

Rules of engagement
Your consultation checklist

- **Does the doctor have hospital privileges, and where?**
  This is a formality, but an essential one. In America, a surgeon should come with a title like 'Attending Surgeon' or 'Assistant Clinical Professor' at some institution, preferably one that you have heard of before. In the UK, there are precious few actual 'Professor' titles to go round, but look for 'Consultant Plastic Surgeon'. Academic titles don't necessarily make up for a lack of aesthetic judgement and skill, but a doctor out of formal training for more than a few years who has not been published in peer-reviewed medical journals should raise suspicions. Your cosmetic surgeon should also maintain an association with at least one or several fully licensed hospitals or clinics.

- **Is the doctor's surgery facility accredited and how long has it been in business?**
  In the UK, doctor's surgeries are required to be licensed by the local health authority, and the documentation should be clearly visible at the location. Freestanding hospitals and clinics require regulation and are subject to frequent inspection according to the standards set forth.

- **What are the risks and complications of the procedure?**
  A reputable doctor will start with the 'D' word (death) and work his way down to infection and bad scars. As horrific as that may sound, all surgery comes with inherent risks. Never tell the doctor that you don't want to know; it is as much your responsibility to find out, as it is his responsibility to inform you. The surgeon has a duty to tell you about complications that occur in more than 1% of the procedures.

- **How long will the procedure take?**
  Surgeons have a natural tendency to downplay the extent of the surgery. They are not always being deliberately misleading; they are just being 'surgeons'. Nothing EVER takes 15 minutes. It will take longer to wheel you into the operating theatre and prep you with anaesthetic. If your surgeon says the procedure will take 6 or more hours, you might want to get a second opinion to see if that amount of time is reasonable for the operation proposed.

- **How long will the results last?**
  This translates into 'when will I need to do it again?' With some procedures, the answer may be 'never', as in breast reductions or nasal surgery. Of course, this will vary from lift to lift as well.

- **How long will I take to heal?**
  This question is impossible to answer with any degree of certainty. No surgeon can promise you that you'll be bruise-free by any given date. A facelift is a process that can take many months to reach its final resting-place, but you should have a general idea.

- **How much time will I have to take off work? When can I drive?**
  Ask your surgeon the above questions to aid you in planning and recruiting available assistants who can drive you to and from the clinic for suture removal and check-ups. The use of dissolving sutures in cosmetic surgery has significantly cut down on stitch and dressing removal visits.

- **What anaesthesia will be given and who will be administering it?**
  In the UK and Australia, only a medical doctor is licensed to administer an anaesthetic, not a nurse. Anaesthetists are medically trained specialists that have to become medical doctors first and then go on to do a minimum of 2–3 years of general training in a hospital. The choice of anaesthetist is often not something you have control over, but it is reasonable to ask to speak with the anaesthetist in advance of surgery. The options of local or general anaesthetic will be discussed with both the anaesthetist and your surgeon.

- **If I don't like the result, what can be done?**
  Surgery is not a perfect science, so make sure your doctor stands behind his work and is willing to do what it takes to make you happy (within reason, of course). Fortunately, most poor surgical outcomes can be improved, at least

to some degree. Know in advance what kind of recourse you might have.

- **What are the alternatives?**
  If you decide not to have the surgery the doctor is recommending, find out what else you can have done instead to improve the feature you are concerned about or what else it might take to make yourself look younger, prettier, softer, etc.

- **If I were your sister/daughter/wife, would you tell me to have the surgery?**
  Look him straight in the eyes when you ask this. It's harder to give a trumped up answer to a direct question like this, but save it for last…

budgeting

One of the first questions I ask my clients is 'Do you have a specific budget in mind?' The reason for this is not because I secretly double as an agent for the Inland Revenue, but rather to try to set some guidelines. Shock is not an uncommon phenomenon in cosmetic surgery. Many have been known to get lightheaded when first presented with a facelift fee quotation. When you base fees on the adverts at the back of the glossies, which claim a nose re-shaping for as low as £150 a month or a facelift in a war-torn republic for £2,500 including airfare and 'deluxe' accommodation, you are bound to be disappointed when private doctor's fees are discussed. If a woman has only £5,000 to spend in total and she wants a facelift, I might recommend doing her lids now and some fat transplants, and saving up for the lift. You don't have to be ashamed to tell the truth about what you can and cannot afford. If you can't quite manage the fees, you might be able to get a recommendation to a more junior colleague whose fees might be lower. If you're pleasant, stable, not neurotic and have realistic expectations, a surgeon might be more willing to work with you or give you a referral.

The doctor who charges the highest fees is also not necessarily the best surgeon. Money is always an issue, even for the rich and famous, but it should never be the overriding factor in your decision. At the end of the day, a few thousand pounds more, amortized out over the lifespan of a facial rejuvenation procedure, amounts to just a few pounds a day. The other consideration is the many thousands of pounds it may cost to correct badly done cosmetic work, that is often more than the fee for the original operation. Quality cosmetic surgery does not come cheap and cheap plastic surgery often proves to be the most dear in the long run. One trick to watch out for is the ubiquitous, 'I just had a cancellation for next Friday, and I'll give you a £1,000 off if you take that date.' If you went to see 3 doctors who are all in the same basic price range for similar procedures (within £1–2,000 or so), and the fourth one you see in the same city is a third less, that should raise a red flag.

If you're thinking about having your face done but aren't sure about the eyes, brow or laser, the 'package' price will always be better value than if you have the face done now, and the eyes done a year from now. You will also not have the additional hospital and anaesthetic fees incurred when you do it in stages. Sometimes a surgeon will throw in something small that won't take him much time, like dermabrasion of the upper lip. If a surgeon is just a bit too eager to cut a deal with you, look out.

It's always better to have a really great eyelift, than a mediocre head-to-toe makeover. The chart on the next page (What does it cost?) will give you a basic idea of what looking younger will cost in major cities where the highest fees prevail. There are many less expensive surgeons and also a small group of celebrity surgeons, whose fees are even higher. Fees are often at least 20% lower in less fashionable cities such as Manchester, Bristol and Birmingham, or Dallas, Philadelphia, Atlanta. Some of the more favourable places in terms of fees are Canada, South Africa, Costa Rica and Scandinavia. The really cheap plastic is in Central America and Eastern Europe; for example, a tuck in Ecuador costs about £1,000, but you might lose some skin in the process.

The fees outlined in the What does it cost? box opposite DO NOT include the costs of a hospital or clinic, the anaesthetist or other incidentals. These are a minimum spend.

What does it cost?

Surgery	London	New York/Los Angeles	Sydney
Eyelids	£3–4,000	$5–8,000	$5–7,000
Facelift	£4–7,000	$8–12,000	$6–9,000
Facelift with eyelids	£6–9,000	$12–18,000	$8–12,000
Total facial rejuvenation (face, eyelids, brow, laser)	£8–12,000	$15–22,000	$10–14,000

Find out in advance what the surgeon's fee will cover. Generally, it will include all of the post-operative follow-up appointments for up to one year after surgery. There are usually separately itemized fees for the surgeon, the anaesthetist and the hospital. Most cosmetic surgeons will expect their full fee to be paid at least two weeks prior to surgery, and some will require an initial deposit to secure a date (up to £500 or 10% of the surgical fee) that may or may not be refundable. Regrettably, your John Lewis Partnership card is not likely to be accepted. The hospital will require payment at the time of admission as well. Surgeons commonly accept major credit cards for payment, debit cards, personal cheques, banker's drafts and, of course, cash, as payment. Credit cards present a great opportunity to rack up airline miles, so you get a free flight as a bonus for having a lift. Some surgeons and clinics may offer a financing option, with a small monthly fee plus sky-high interest over a three-year period equivalent to rates previously only charged by Reggie Kray. Generally, it is not a good idea to go into hock for a facelift. However, if your face is your fortune, you have to expect it to cost you a fortune too. Facial rejuvenation procedures are one time you want to pay retail. As Christina Carlino, of BioMedic Clinical Skincare says, 'When it comes to making an incision on your face, do not shop price. Shop qualifications.'

how to tell the pros from the cons
– traps to avoid

There is a sharp distinction between 'bad' doctors and doctors who just aren't very good – the surgeon who cuts corners or does sloppy work; the surgeon who has lost his touch; the surgeon who throws instruments in the operating theatre; or the surgeon who is stuck in a time-warp and refuses to even consider improved methods because 'we've been doing it this way for years'. They should all be avoided. In medicine, difficulties may arise without warning and it requires fortitude to take whatever comes your way. Surgeons are supposed to be tougher, steadier and better equipped in temperament to handle the pressures than mere mortals; after all, the rigours of medical training are designed to weed out the weaker ones.

The sad fact is that when a doctor's judgement takes a frequent turn for the worse, the medical establishment and the powers that be are almost entirely unequipped to do anything about it at all. It is often a matter of years before effective action can be enforced against a 'bad' doctor, however hazardous he may be to women's faces. The people who are in the best position to see firsthand how dangerous a doctor may be are arguably in the worst position to do anything to stop it, for example registrars, nurses and surgical assistants. A prospective patient would be wise to treat an endorsement like, 'He's a good doctor, but sometimes he has his moments', with appropriate caution.

Beware of doctors who present a prepared list of references. That's fine when you're enlisting someone to patch your roof, but stock testimonials offer little value and you can't be sure that the referee isn't the surgeon's sister-in-law. Don't allow yourself to get pressed into doing more surgery than you really want; too little is better than too much and you can always do more later on. There are advantages to doing a facelift with eyelid surgery at the same time, but when you start fooling around with too many areas at once, you may feel overwhelmed. Generally, it is safer to do face work together, and body work at another stage, rather than combining it all at once.

Be very wary of websites, mailers, brochures, videos and adverts with tarty half-dressed women, or promises of discounts and bargains. These are not the most reliable ways to find a surgeon. Make sure your surgeon will be around if you have a problem. If it sounds too good to be true in cosmetic surgery, it definitely is.

Better shop around

Top reasons patients get put off by doctors:

- Cold and 'impersonal' treatment
  Can't 'connect' with surgeon – 'too distant', 'doesn't seem interested', 'didn't listen'
- Too aggressive approach
  'Wants to do too much'
- Too conservative approach
  'Won't do enough'
- Lack of confidence in the surgeon
- Felt 'rushed' or 'pressured'
- The consulting rooms seemed like a 'factory'
- The doctor refused to show any photos of his work
- Hasn't seen anyone the doctor has operated on
- Has seen someone doctor operated on and didn't like the result
- Too long to wait – for appointment, for surgery, to see the doctor, etc
- Doesn't seem up to date on new techniques
- Made the surgery seem too radical
  'You'll have a scar behind your ear like an appendix scar...'
- He didn't listen, pay attention or take notes
- Over-promises
  'You're going to look like your younger sister when I get done with you'
- Condescending tone and criticisms
  'You don't have great bones'
- Suggesting a surgery unrelated to what you're interested in
  'We can fix up your nose at the same time...'
- Seductive manner and asking questions that border on too personal
- Discussed another patient with you
  'I'd just die if he told someone I had my face done'

According to Professor David T. Sharpe, OBE, Past President of the British Association of Aesthetic Plastic Surgeons, 'Patients must remember that there is a strong commercial imperative for clinics to sell an operation, whether the patient needs it or not. They work on the basis that by advertising and employing doctors to perform a large number of cases at a relatively cheap rate, a handsome profit can be made. The best action is to go only to a named practitioner whose reputation is vital to maintaining his practice.' Regrettably, many patients are vulnerable to seduction by unscrupulous surgeons in search of any patient with a cheque book. There are many valid reasons for walking away, and often they are based on gut instinct. If it doesn't feel right, keep looking until you find a surgeon who makes you feel comfortable and whom you have faith in.

The great lies in cosmetic surgery
'I'm the only one doing this procedure'
'I've never had a complication'
'I do more of these than anyone else'
'I invented this operation'
'I fix everyone else's mistakes'
'He learned it from me'
'You'll only feel a little pinch'
'You'll be a little red for a few days'
'You won't even see the scars'
'No one does it that way any more'
'Of course it won't hurt'
'You will be astonished at the improvement'
'It's cheaper than you think'
'It's going to be just perfect'
'Just two treatments will be more than enough'
'It will put a fresh spark into your love life'
'I do all the models and film stars'

complications and other misfortunes of surgery

Your risks of surgical complications increase exponentially with age, health status and physical condition. For example, a heart condition, hypertension, diabetes or obesity will not necessarily disqualify you for a facelift operation, but it will definitely factor into how much surgery you can safely have done at one stage. Luckily, the rate of complications from well-executed facial cosmetic surgery is very low. The list below indicates the most common risks, and the average incidence of each.

Top complications of facelifting

Haematoma	3%
Hair-loss	1%
Skin-loss	1%
Poor scars	1.5%
Infections	0.5%
Facial nerve damage	0.025%

(SOURCE: Barry M. Jones, FRCS)

Haematoma
A possible complication of any surgery is a haematoma, or collection of blood under the skin that may or may not have to be reopened and drained. These range from tiny little collections that will resolve on their own, to dense areas of bleeding that will necessitate going back to the operating theatre. Smokers, people with high blood pressure and men are often more prone to haematoma. If you are too active following surgery, you also increase your chances of having one.

Hair loss
According to Mr Barry Jones, 'Permanent hair loss following a facelift will only occur if there is too much tension put on the hair-bearing

skin or the vector of the lift is incorrect. I always ask women considering a facelift about their hairstyle and particularly whether they wear their hair "up". Most women should be able to wear their hair in any style they choose after a facelift, providing the scars are placed appropriately. If they do like to wear their hair "up" it is sensible to leave it a little softer behind the ears and not to scrape it up too severely during the initial healing phase of 4–6 weeks.'

Skin loss

A haematoma left untreated can result in skin 'necrosis' or slough. If there is not a rich enough blood supply at a surgical site, the skin may become dark, blackened and eventually scab and fall off. This may leave a discoloured area in the skin or a displeasing scar that requires attention.

Poor scars

Raised, thickened, red, angry or over-exuberant scars can sometimes occur after cosmetic surgery, and will settle down over time. Lasers can be used to reduce pigment in scars, and raised scars can be made flatter. Scars that mature into white, flat, widened and stretched patches are the most difficult to improve without excising or cutting out the actual scar tissue. According to Dr Mendelson, 'Scars in younger people do not heal as well as in older people. This may seem paradoxical but it is a significant fact in cosmetic facial surgery.'

Infections

Infections are rare, but have to be treated immediately to avoid more serious problems and spread. Incisions must be kept clean and you will be instructed to keep your hands off. Most surgeons will provide antibiotic therapy at some point (before, during, after) during the course of your surgery to guard against infection.

Facial nerve damage

The incidence of permanent facial nerve damage is luckily quite low. Some numbness is normal following face and browlift surgery. On rare occasions, one of the facial nerves may display a weakness immediately after surgery. Transient nerve injuries will usually resolve on their own within 6 months as the swelling goes down, although there is never a guarantee. Clearly, this is one example of when skill and an in-depth knowledge of facial anatomy is paramount in your surgeon.

According to Mr Waterhouse, most of the complications of browlifting, such as itching, numbness, headaches and hair loss, are also transient: 'In a very small number of patients, there can be a paralysis of the frontal branch which causes a weakness of raising one brow. If too much of the muscles in the glabella are resected, a depression can result which may need a graft placed to make it smooth,' he says, adding, 'eighty-five per cent of all patients who have had an endoscopic browlift would recommend it to a friend.'

what to do if it goes horribly wrong

If your original face-, eyelid- or browlift was not properly done, you may be forced to wait until the tissues loosen up sufficiently before you can be re-operated on. It takes from 6 months to a year before the healing process is complete. The first anniversary is usually the earliest point at which you should contemplate going under the knife again. If you are still unhappy after you have healed completely, analyze what exactly you are dissatisfied with.

Telltale signs of bad work
- Upper eyelids won't close all the way
- Pulled down lower eyelids (scleral show)
- Raised hairline at the temples
- Tunnels or dents in the lower cheeks
- Distorted ear shape, attached earlobes
- Pleating or skin bunching
- 'Fish mouth'
- Eyelids that look too pointy or too sad

- Hollowed out eyelids
- Thickened red scars behind the ears
- Widened or stretched whitened scars in the hairline
- Marked asymmetries or unevenness (one side higher or lower or bigger)
- Badly positioned scars
- Stitch marks visible
- Pixie ears

Ask a friend to take a good look at you and get an honest opinion. Consult with your GP or dermatologist for their opinions on whether your lift was properly done. There is a fine line between whether your expectations going into surgery were reasonable or highly inflated. The other consideration is whether your hopes and aspirations of youthful perfection were in fact the result of your own misunderstanding or the fault of the surgeon in not explaining it well. Most of the time, it is a function of a lack of communication between the doctor and the patient. As Dr Guy Jost advises, 'If you have a result in mind from a facelift, you should divide it in half.' Unless you have lost confidence in the original surgeon, you should go back and see him again to discuss your feelings with him directly. If your surgeon agrees that the result is not as good as it should be, a reputable surgeon may be willing to revise it at a reduced fee or at no charge. Hospital fees and charges for the anaesthetist may be incurred, however. Find out what recourse is open to you if you are unhappy with the results, for example if there are limitations as to what can be done, what the risks of further scarring are and whether there is a likelihood that you will be happy after a second procedure. The risks with each subsequent procedure increase proportionally.

One of the greatest fears women have about undergoing cosmetic surgery is that they are stuck if it goes wrong. Most results can be improved by additional revisionary surgery and/or the passage of time. There is a wide range of reactions that often accompany a dissatisfying surgical result that include embarrassment, guilt, blame, rage, shame and disappointment. Many women are most angry at themselves for having chosen poorly. The 'I should have known better', 'I shouldn't have listened' and 'How could I have been so stupid' responses are common. The guilt comes when an unsupportive spouse or mate reminds you, 'It serves you right for going to fool around with what nature gave you'. This flurry of emotions ends up being a colossal waste of time. What's done is done, and it is healthier to just move on.

There are many cases when having a secondary procedure will only heighten your state of anxiety, and a cooling down period before you go ahead is wiser. If you find yourself slipping into a depression, it may be time to seek intervention from a professional counsellor or psychotherapist.

English women may often consider an untoward result somehow acceptable and even respectable to some degree, and are far less likely than demanding New Yorkers to make a fuss about it. Your first step should never be to visit your solicitor. Bringing litigation in the courts against a surgeon is a gruelling process for all parties involved (except perhaps the lawyers) and serves little purpose other than pure revenge. The threat of a lawsuit will immediately shut down your relationship with the surgeon and may also discourage other surgeons from getting involved with you if they fear that you will drag them into court. Taking legal action is always the last resort and doesn't solve the problem of an unsatisfactory surgical result. Neither does the longstanding British tradition of writing to the papers.

Success in cosmetic surgery can only be measured by whether the patient is satisfied; the doctor's opinion is basically irrelevant. According to Dr John Celin, 'The practice of cosmetic surgery is an inexact art. You can't expect to get a guarantee of the exact result you want or any warranty against an unwanted result.'

Five possible cosmetic surgery outcomes
- Both the patient and the surgeon are happy.
- The surgeon is happy, but the patient isn't.
- The patient is happy, but the surgeon isn't.
- The patient can never be happy.
- The surgeon can never be happy.

afterword

New technologies are now emerging into the field of cosmetic surgery as fast as dot com companies. In the first decade of the 21st century, we can expect to witness the impact of microchips and nanosurgery on facelifting. The buzzwords to pay attention to are: telesurgery, genetic engineering, the human genome project, voice-controlled robotic manipulators, 3-D stereo endoscopes, mechanically-assisted surgery and lasers that target diseased tissues with pinpoint accuracy. New advances among tools for diagnosis and treatment in medicine will filter down into plastic surgery, dermatology and dentistry. These developments, coupled with the growing acceptance of the Internet as a source for health and medicine information, will revolutionize the profession, and reduce the barriers that many women are faced with when they think about doing something to their wrinkles and bags.

Ideas and discoveries can now be shared at a much faster rate between specialists across cities, countries and continents. Although the science and technology aspects are more than my liberal arts education has prepared me to absorb at once, I welcome it on with open arms and deepening lines. Anything that holds the promise of downsizing recovery times, bruising, swelling and the length and visibility of scars over the coming years is all right with me, as long as it is also safe and effective. On top of my wish list for the future is that cosmetic surgery won't always cost a fortune so that more women could do what they want when they want it, rather than having to save up for an eternity. It seems only fair that women should be given a new face and body for their 30th birthdays, when they have finally grown to respect their bodies and learned to care for them properly.

In the meantime though, I'm checking my diary for a window of time to have a little tweaking of my own done in the coming months. I am often reminded of one very ancient punchline, 'If I knew I was going to live this long, I would have taken better care of myself...'

The most exciting aspect of the field of aesthetic medicine is that it is constantly evolving and represents an endless series of learning curves. You never know what's coming next.

What's your maintenance IQ?

Take our Multiple Choice Personal Assessment and find out how you really feel about your appearance.

1. You've laddered your best pair of tights, so you:
a) Do nothing and wait until you get home
b) Keep pulling your skirt hem down to cover the offending snag
c) Dash into Selfridge's for an emergency replacement pair

2. Your last pedicure was:
a) Never
b) Can't remember
c) A few weeks ago

3. Your holiday to Spain is one week away. What's on your mind?:
a) He's working late tonight so I can borrow his shaver
b) Get out the pot of wax and turn on the stove
c) Call to get squeezed in for a laser touch-up ASAP

4. You would never leave home without:
a) An emery board
b) Lip balm
c) A fully-stocked makeup kit

5. The foundation you've been using since discontinued, so you:
a) Wipe the sweat dripping from your brow as you log on to Prozac.com
b) Flip through the glossies for what Minnie, Nicole and Gwyneth are wearing
c) Ring up all 103 branches of John Lewis to buy up every last one in stock

6. Your reaction to reading that your skin is being attacked by free radicals is:
a) At least they're free so no one is charging me
b) You run out to slather on the SPF50
c) You cancel your dinner date and stay home through summer

7. Your sister-in-law remarks over tea that your lipstick is bleeding into the lines above your lip. You:
a) Pat your mouth with your napkin
b) Excuse yourself and run to the powder room for repairs
c) Pull out your mobile and call the clinic for an emergency collagen shot

8. You're walking past the window of Harvey Nick's and spy a spot right on the tip of your nose. You:
a) Look away and shrug your shoulders
b) Recoil in horror and dash to the nearest Boot's for some anti-spot gel pronto
c) Pull out your industrial strength cream makeup to cover the eruption

9. How many lipsticks do you really need?
a) One or two
b) One for every day of the week
c) You can never be too rich, too thin or have too many lipsticks

10. The only available appointment with your colourist is next week and you've got roots for days. You:
a) Risk it
b) Invest a small fortune in hair accessories to deflect attention from your dark roots
c) Beg, plead, and whimper until you get squeezed in this week

11. You read about a new miracle cream in Vogue that's touted to smooth your crows feet. You:
a) Turn the page because your lines aren't really that bad
b) Clip out the article and tuck it in your dresser drawer for safe keeping
c) Phone the stockist and place an order straight away before they sell out

What's your maintenance IQ? – The answers
Total up your As, Bs, and Cs and then read on.

Mostly A's:
LOW MAINTENANCE

Your approach to grooming is that you can't be bothered. You prefer short-term, simple and temporary solutions that require little or no effort on your part, rather than anything fussy or complicated. Your image conveys who you are and where you came from: solid, reliable and a believer in function above form.

You are happy with the way you look and have never entertained dreams of becoming a raving beauty. You resolutely reject society's view of how a woman should look and any state-enforced ideal of beauty. As for beauty fixes, you can take them or leave them. You might have a facial and get talked into trying one or two CACI treatments or linger at the moisturizers aisle at Tesco out of idle curiosity, but you are seldom inclined to take it that one step further. It goes against your very nature to even consider changing a God-given feature or erasing a wrinkle, and you are often heard to say, 'I've had this face my whole life and I've grown rather fond of it.' And we all know that true beauty emanates from within.

Mostly B's:
MIDDLE MAINTENANCE

After careful introspection, you realize that you could easily be persuaded to become more concerned with your outward appearance if given a gentle nudge. You are comfortable in your own skin, but strive to preserve what you've got, or even to better it. There is also a secret, vampish side to you that you reveal to only your closest friends, and you have been known to indulge in the occasional frills, adornments and hedonistic delights.

If your great-aunt suddenly passed and left you a tidy inheritance, you might be tempted to splurge some of it on some surgical intervention, but you remain reasonably sceptical of the outcome. You have some lingering guilt about spending your precious hard-earned money on things as frivolous as your looks, but you are intrigued by glitz and glam. A trigger event such as your husband having an affair with someone at the office, or your son's engagement, or the grand opening of a Wrinkle Clinic across the road could push you right over the edge.

Mostly C's:

HIGH MAINTENANCE

You have clearly graduated right up the ranks and made it to a respectable level. You may not yet have achieved the necessary financial allowance to accomplish all of your beauty goals, but the flesh is willing and your heart is definitely in it. With some encouragement, you are dangling close to full-fledged Beauty Junkie status. Of particular appeal to you is the notion of gently improving on what Mother Nature doled out to you in the first place, and hanging on to it for dear life. No price is too high to pay for anything than can further those goals and no sacrifice too great. You read with great zeal about the latest trends in cutting-edge cosmetic treatments, innovations and surgical enhancements, and wonder how it is that Goldie Hawn looks the same today as she did in 1975. You take great joy in sharing your wisdom on these matters with others, and begin avoiding birthdays and lying about when you went to university. As your inquisitiveness starts nagging at you, you find yourself staring at every pretty face you come across to see 'what she's had done'.

Final countdown – 1,2,3, lift-off...

Here's a guide to planning for your surgery. Remember, preparation is all and has a tremendous effect on the final outcome of your surgery. If you want the best results, get prepared.

1 month before

☐ Go for your pre-operative blood tests, ECG, X-ray
☐ Have your last visit to the hairdresser before surgery, keeping your hair long around the ears
☐ Have a deep cleansing facial
☐ Start an active anti-ageing vitamin A,E,C-enriched skincare regime
☐ OTHER

3 weeks before

☐ Stop all aspirin and other drugs that cause bleeding. Stop taking Vitamin E
☐ Avoid multi-vitamins and natural supplements
☐ Stop smoking and/or taking nicotine substitutes
☐ OTHER

2 weeks before

☐ If requested, discontinue HRT
☐ Load up on Vitamin C (1000 mg/day)
☐ Cut down on wine and spirits
☐ OTHER

1 week before

☐ Last chance for highlights or colouring your hair
☐ Pick up a camouflage cream and green undertone cream for concealing bruises
☐ Get supplies from the pharmacy (gloves, gauzes, hydrogen peroxide, swabs, etc.)
☐ Have your prescriptions for pain medication filled if you've been given them
☐ Have a Manual Lymphatic Drainage treatment to eliminate toxins
☐ Get your brows waxed or plucked
☐ OTHER

The day before
- [ ] Stock your fridge with broth, juices, water, teas, soft foods
- [ ] Pack your hospital bag with nightie, slippers, toothbrush
- [ ] Start your Arnica tablets or capsules, if requested
- [ ] Begin your antibiotics, if prescribed
- [ ] Buy a good book or your favourite magazines and rent a few videos
- [ ] Call your surgeon's secretary to confirm the time to arrive at hospital
- [ ] Schedule your first post-op visit to the surgeon
- [ ] OTHER

The night before
- [ ] Remove nail lacquer, if requested, and contact lenses
- [ ] Set your alarm
- [ ] Enjoy a leisurely dinner with your husband/partner/friend, avoiding alcohol or highly salted and spiced foods
- [ ] Wash your hair twice
- [ ] Have nothing to eat or drink after midnight
- [ ] Fill all the ice trays in the freezer
- [ ] OTHER

The morning of the surgery
- [ ] Wear loose-fitting clothes and nothing that pulls over your head
- [ ] Wash your face and brush your teeth
- [ ] Don't apply moisturiser, fragrance or makeup
- [ ] Change the bed linens to old ones and fluff your pillows
- [ ] Arrange your bedside tray with everything you will need
- [ ] Leave your jewellery and wristwatch at home
- [ ] OTHER

Your personal medical history

Photocopy and then complete this form before you take it along with you to your consultations. This will help you inform your surgeon about all your relevant medical details and make sure that you don't leave anything out

Name ———————————————————————————————

Date of Birth ————————————————————————————

Age ————————————————————————————————

Height ————————————————————————————————

Weight ————————————————————————————————

Name of GP ————————————————————————————

Address ————————————————————————————————

Telephone ———————————————————————————————

Facsimile ————————————————————————————————

List all previous surgery with dates

Operation	Date	Surgeon

Have you had an adverse reaction to:

- ☐ Anaesthestic
- ☐ Antibiotics
- ☐ Codeine
- ☐ Demerol

- ☐ Adhesive tape
- ☐ Aspirin
- ☐ Sulphur
- ☐ Penicillin

- ☐ Valium
- ☐ Iodine
- ☐ Morphine
- ☐ Suture material

Do you have a history of:

- ☐ Diabetes
- ☐ Asthma
- ☐ Bleeding disorders
- ☐ Cancer
- ☐ Keloid or
     hypertrophic scars
- ☐ Excessive bruising
- ☐ Bronchitis, chronic
     cough
- ☐ Tuberculosis
- ☐ Radiotherapy

- ☐ Hernia
- ☐ Shortness of breath
- ☐ Hypertension
- ☐ Blood clots
- ☐ Headaches
- ☐ Cold sores, Herpes
- ☐ Hepatitis A, B or C
- ☐ Mitral valve prolapse,
     Heart murmur
- ☐ Drug abuse
- ☐ Alcoholism

- ☐ Nose bleeds
- ☐ Thyroid problems
- ☐ Dry eye
- ☐ Seizures
- ☐ Depression
- ☐ Facial paralysis
- ☐ Osteo or Rheumatoid
     arthritis
- ☐ Lupus or Auto-Immune
     Disease
- ☐ Other

Have you taken:

- ☐ Blood pressure
     medication
- ☐ Cardiac medication
- ☐ Diet pills
- ☐ Diuretics
- ☐ Vitamin, mineral and
     herbal supplements

- ☐ Tranquilizers
- ☐ Alcohol
- ☐ Sleeping pills
- ☐ Anti-depressants
- ☐ Pain medication
- ☐ Roaccutane
- ☐ HRT

- ☐ Aspririn or other
     anti-inflammatories

Do you have any allergies to medications? If so, list them here:

Diary of a consultation

Doctor _____

Tel _____

Consulting rooms _____

Secretary/Nurse _____

Diagnosis (the doctor's findings)

```
┌──────────────────────────────────────────────┐
│                                                │
│                                                │
│                                                │
│                                                │
│                                                │
└──────────────────────────────────────────────┘
```

Treatment plan (tick all that apply)

☐ BOTOX
☐ Fat transfer
☐ Liposuction of the neck
☐ Lower lid fat removal
☐ Upper lid skin, fat removal
☐ Endoscopic browlift
☐ Open forehead lift
☐ Temporal or upper facelift
☐ Midface lift or cheeklift
☐ OTHER

☐ Lip augmentation
☐ Chin implant
☐ Lower facelift
☐ Endoscopic facelift
☐ Face and necklift
☐ Composite facelift
☐ Subperiosteal lift
☐ Resurfacing – Erbium:YAG
☐ Resurfacing – Carbon Dioxide

Procedure performed (tick)

☐ In hospital   ☐ Day case   ☐ Doctor's surgery

Name of hospital _____

Anaesthetic (tick)

☐ Local   ☐ Twilight   ☐ General

Fees

Surgeon _____   Implants _____

Anaesthetist _____   OTHER _____

Hospital _____   TOTAL: _____

Photos (tick)

☐ taken   ☐ to be arranged

Methods of payment (tick)

☐ credit card   ☐ debit card   ☐ cheque   ☐ cash

Lead time for surgery date (tick)

☐ up to 4 weeks   ☐ 4-8 weeks   ☐ 8-12 weeks
☐ 3-6 months   ☐ 6 months+

Deposit amount _____

Deposit due _____

Balance due _____

Notes

Rating your surgeon

1 = Awful   2 = Not so good   3 = Just OK   4 = Very good   5 = Excellent

Calling the office	1	2	3	4	5
Making the appointment	1	2	3	4	5
Wait to see doctor	1	2	3	4	5
Time spent with doctor	1	2	3	4	5
Listening skills and patience	1	2	3	4	5
Instilled confidence and comfort	1	2	3	4	5
Sensible recommendations	1	2	3	4	5
Patient education materials	1	2	3	4	5
Explained surgery & details	1	2	3	4	5
Pressure or pushiness of staff	1	2	3	4	5

Scores from 10-50

Scoring

You're looking for a score of 40 or better, which calculates into 80 per cent. If you have seen the same surgeon more than once, score your visit a second time and calculate the average of the two scores.

For example: 1st score   = 32
2nd score   = 42

Total   = 74 divided by 2
Final Score   = 37

Would you use this surgeon? (tick)

Yes   No   Maybe

Medical societies & resources

UK

The British Association of Aesthetic Plastic Surgeons
Royal College of Surgeons
35-43 Lincoln's Inn Fields
London WC2A 3PN
www.baaps.org.uk

The British Association of Plastic Surgeons
Royal College of Surgeons
35-43 Lincoln's Inn Fields
London WC2A 3PN
T: (+44) 020 7831 5161
www.baps.co.uk

The British Association of Dermatologists
19 Fitzroy Square
London WC1H 5HQ
T: (+44) 020 7383 0266
E-mail address: admin@bad.org.uk
www.bad.org.uk/index.cfm

The Department of Health
Alert line 0800 004440
Information Service 0800 665544
Freephone info line 0800 216 613

Medicines Control Agency (MCA)
Market Towers
1 Nine Elms Lane
London SW8 5NQ
T: (+44) 020 7273 0000
F: (+44) 020 7273 0353

The British Medical Association
BMA House
Tavistock Square
London WC1H 9JP
T: (+44) 020 7387 4499

The Royal College of Ophthalmologists
17 Cornwall Terrace
London NW1 4QW
T: (+44) 020 7935 0702
www.rcophth.ac.uk

The General Medical Council
178-202 Great Portland Street
London W1N 6AE
T: (+44) 020 7580 7642
E-mail address: gmc@gmc-uk.org
www.gmc-uk.org
The GMC is the registering body for doctors and is able to help advise on doctors' qualifications.

Patient Association
PO Box 935
Harrow
Middlesex HA1 3YJ
T: (+44) 020 423 8999
F: (+44) 020 423 9119

Royal College of Anaesthetists
48-49 Russell Square
London WC1B 4JY
T: (+44) 0207908 7300
F: (+44) 020 7813 1876
Info@rcoa.ac.uk
www.rcoa.ac.uk

Association of Anaesthetists
9 Bedford Square
London WC1B 3RE
T: (+44) 020 7631 1650
F. (+44) 020 7631 4352
www.aagbi.org

AUSTRALIA

**Australian Society
of Plastic Surgeons**
Level 1, 33-35 Atchinson Street
St Leonards 2065 NSW Australia
Tel: 61 2 9437 9200
Fax: 61 2 9437 9210
www.asps.asn.au

**Australasian College
of Dermatologists**
PO Box B65 Boronia Park
NSW 2111 Australia
T: 61 02 9879 6177
F: 61 02 9816 1174
austcollderm@bigpond.com

NEW ZEALAND

**New Zealand Association of Plastic
Reconstructive Aesthetic Surgeons**
Tristram Plastic Surgery and
Dermatology Group
103 Tristram Street
Hamilton
New Zealand
T: (64) 7 838 1035
F: (64) 7 838 2032

New Zealand Dermatological Society
www.demnet.org.nz

SOUTH AFRICA

**Association of Plastic and
Reconstructive Surgeons
of Southern Africa**
PO Box 130891
PO Box 3151
Bryanston 2021
Republic of South Africa
Tel: (27) 11463 1210
Fax: (27) 11463 2485
www.plasticsurgeons.co.za

UNITED STATES

**American Society
for Aesthetic Plastic Surgery**
11081 Winners Circle, Suite 200
Los Alamitos, California 90720
www.surgery.org
*The leading organization of plastic
surgeons certified by the American
Board of Plastic Surgery (or the Royal
College of Physicians and Surgeons of
Canada) who specialize in cosmetic
surgery of the face and body.*

American Society of Plastic Surgeons
444 E. Algonquin Road
Arlington Heights, IL 60005
www.surgery.org
*Represents physicians certified by the
American Board of Plastic Surgery
(ABPS) or the Royal College of
Physicians and Surgeons of Canada.*

American Academy of Dermatology
930 N. Meacham Road
Schaumburg, IL 60168-4014
www.aad.org
*The largest and most representative of
all dermatologic associations, with over
13,000 dermatologists worldwide.*

**American Academy of Facial Plastic
and Reconstructive Surgery**
310 S. Henry Street
Alexandria, Virginia 22314
www.aafprs.org

**The American Society for
Dermatologic Surgery**
930 N. Meacham Road
Schaumburg, IL 60173-6016
www.asds-net.org
asds@neton-line.com
*Promotes excellence in
dermatologic surgery.*

INTERNATIONAL

**International Plastic and
Reconstructive Association**
www.ipras.org
*If you are looking for a surgeon in
a country other than those listed
here, this site has a complete listing
of plastic surgical societies in all
countries, with contact information.*

**European Academy of Dermatology
and Venereology**
www.eadv.org
*If you are looking for a dermatologist
or dermatologic surgeon in Europe
or outside of Europe, this site has a
complete listing of plastic surgical
societies in all countries.*

International Society of Dermatology
930 N. Meacham Road
Schaumburg, IL 60173-6016
T: 847-330-9830
F: 847-330-1135
www.intsocdermatol.org

Physician sources

My sincere thanks to the following physicians who are quoted in the book. I wish I could list all the others I interviewed and visited as well, but space limits prevail.

Dr Tina Alster
2311 M Street NW,
Suite 200, Washington DC
20037, USA
T: 001-202-785-8855,
talster@skinlaser.com

Ms Lena Andersson
Anelca Clinic
27 Devonshire Place
London WIN 1PD
T: (+44) 020 7224 4333
anelca@anelca.com

Dr Fritz E. Barton
411 North Washington
Dallas, TX 75246, USA
T: 001-214-821-9355
febart@onramp.net

**Dr Alistair and
Dr Jean Carruthers**
820 943 West Broadway,
Vancouver,
BC V5Z 4E1 Canada
T: 001-604-714-0222
carruth@interchange.ubc.ca

Dr Anita R. Cela
212 E 68th Street
New York, NY 10021
T: 001-212-535-6004

Dr John Celin
34 Hans Road
London SW3 1RW
T: (+44) 020 7225 0179
jcelin@compuserve.com

**Dr Bernard Cornette
de Saint Cyr**
15 Rue de Spontini
Paris, 75116, France
T: 33 01 47 04 25 02

Brian Coghlan, FRCS
14 Devonshire Mews West,
London
T: (+44) 020 7499 7527

Dr Peter Bela Fodor
2080 Century Park East,
Suite 710, Los Angeles,
CA 90067, USA
T: 001-310-203-9818,
pbfodor@aol.com

Dr Peter Forrester
Peter.forrester@virgin.net

Dr Sam T. Hamra
2731 Lemmon Avenue,
Dallas, TX 75204, USA
T: 001-214-754-9001
drhamra@drhamra.com

**Dr Susan Horsewood-Lee
MB BS MRCGP**
34 Oakley Street,
London SW3 5NT
drsusan@dircon.co.uk,
www:chelseadoctor.com

Barry M. Jones, FRCS
14a Upper Wimpole Street,
London W1M 7TB
T: (+44) 020 7935 1938,
bmjones@globalnet.co.uk

Dr Guy Jost
55 rue de Prony
Paris, 75017, France
T: 33 01 42 22 48 44

Dr Z. Paul Lorenc
983 Park Avenue,
New York, NY 10028
T: 001-212-472-2900,
lorenc@lorenc.com

Professor Nicholas Lowe
The Cranley Clinic
19a Cavendish Square
London W1M 9AD
T: (+44) 020 7499 3223

Mr Andrew Clive Markey
The Lister Hospital
Chelsea Bridge Road
London SW1W 8RH
T: (+44) 020 7730 1219

Dr Alan Matarasso
1009 Park Avenue
New York. NY 10021, USA
T: 001-212-249-7500,
matarasso@aol.com

Dr Seth Matarasso
490 Post Street
Suite 700, San Francisco
CA 94102, USA
T: 001-415-362-2238

Basim A. Matti, FRCS
Flat 2, 30 Harley Street
London W1N 1AB
T: (+44) 020 7637 9595
basimmatti@btconnect.com

Bryan Mendelson, FRCAS
109 Mathoura Road,
Toorak, Melbourne 3142
T: 613 9826 0977
bcm@bmendelson.com.au

Dr Daniel C. Morello
10 Chester Avenue
White Plains
NY 10601, USA
T: 001-914-761-8667
nipntuck@earthlink.net

Mr Gavin Morrison
209 Newlands Surgical Clinic
Main Road
7700 Claremont
South Africa
T: 27 21 689 55 87
Morrison@netactive.co.ca

Keith L. A. Mutimer, FRACS
206 New Street
Brighton 3186
Victoria, Australia
T: 03 9592 0522
kmutimer@asps.asn.au

Dr Foad Nahai
Paces Plastic Surgery
3200 Downwood Circle
Suite 640
Atlanta, GA 30327 USA
T: 001-404-351-0051,
nahaimd@aol.com

Dr Sheldon Pinnell
Duke University Medical
Center, Box 3135
Durham, NC 27710, USA
T: 001-919-684-3002
Sheldon.pinnell@duke.edu

Professor David E. Sharpe
The Yorkshire Clinic
Bradford Road, Bingley
West Yorkshire BD16 1TW
T: (+44) 0127 456 0311

Dr Frank Trepsat
130 Chemin des Fontanieres
Saint-Foy-le-Lyon 69110
France
T: 33 01 78 59 26 79
ftrepsat@asi.fr

Dr David Veale
The Priory Hospital
The Bourne
London N14 6RA
T: (+44) 020 8882 8191,
david@veale.co.uk

**Norman Waterhouse,
FRCS**
55 Harley Street
London W1N 1DD
T: (+44) 020 7636 4073
wtrhouse@globalnet.net

Dr Patricia Wexler
145 East 32nd Street
New York, NY 10016 USA
001-212-684-2626

Dr Donald Wood-Smith
830 Park Avenue
New York NY 10021 USA
T: 001-212-744-2224

Stockists – Major brands mentioned throughout the book (Lancôme, Estée Lauder, Olay, etc) can be found at your local pharmacy and department stores. However, others may be harder to find.

Astara Conscious Skincare – astara.com
Biomedic Clinical Skincare – biomedic.com
Bliss – blissword.com
Caudalie – caudalie.com
Cellex-C – cellex-c.com, (+44) 01342 315892
Chantecaille – at Space NK (+44) 0870 169 9999
Darphin Skincare – at Harrod's (+44) 020 7730 1234, darphinfrance@cs.com
Dr Hauschka – drhauschka.com
Eve Lom – evelom.co.uk, (+44) 020 7935 9988
Home Recovery Cosmetic Surgery Comfort Products – homerecovery.com, 001 843 559 5758
Imedeen (Ferrosan Ltd) – (+44) 020 7240 2122
Jan Marini Skin Research – janmarini.co.uk
Jane Iredale The Skin Care Make Up – janeiredale.com, 0800 349 4444
Joey New York – joeyny.com
Jurlique – jurlique.co.uk, (+44) 020 8841 6644
Kanebo – at Harrod's (+44) 01635 46362
Karin Herzog Skinformation – karinherzog.com
Kinerase (ICN Pharmaceuticals) – icnpharm.com
La Prairie – laprairie.com
Lierac – at Harrod's (+44) 020 7730 1234
Liz Earle Naturally Active Skincare – lizearle.com, (+44) 070 7978 5615
MD Forte – mdformulations.com
Molton Brown – moltonbrown.com, (+44) 020 7911 0070
Neostrata – neostrata.com
Osmotics – osmotics.com
Philosophy – philosophystore.com
Samuel Par – samuelpar.co.uk
Shu Uemura – shuuemura.co.uk
Sisley – sisley.tm.fr, (+44) 020 7591 4466
Skinceuticals – skinceuticals.com
Sothys – sothys.com
Vincent Longo – vincentlongo.com, (+44) 01252 742801

Order your personal subscription to **WLBeauty Watch**

Up-to-the-minute news about cosmetic surgery trends, innovative procedures, post-operative products, interviews with surgeons, and industry scuttlebutt.

The Unofficial Guide to Cosmetic Surgery

Essential for any woman contemplating cosmetic plastic surgery.

Jo Fairley in the *Daily Mail*, YOU Magazine

First name ————————————————————————————

Last name ————————————————————————————

Address ————————————————————————————

Country ————————————————————————————

Postal code ————————————————————————————

Email ————————————————————————————

Phone ————————————————————————————

Card No ————————————————————————————

Exp Date ————————————————————————————

Credit Card   ☐ Visa   ☐ Mastercard   ☐ American Express

(Sorry, Debit cards cannot be accepted at this time)

£25.00 within the UK, £30.00 outside the UK (Only British sterling is accepted)

Mail or fax credit card information or cheque to:
Wendy Lewis
at 15 Sloane Gardens, London SW1W 8EB UK
T/F: 0870 7430 544
Subscription orders can also be placed online at www.wlbeauty.com

Glossary

Ablation
Vaporization of the most superficial layers of skin.

Acne
Chronic condition characterized by an inflammatory eruption of the skin.

Allograft
A graft from the same species as the recipient.

Anaesthetic
A drug that causes a loss of sensation.

Arnica
A botanical derived from a mountain plant with antiseptic, astringent, antimicrobial and anti-inflammatory properties.

Asymmetry
Differences in the two sides of the face or in individual parts of the face that are in pairs, e.g. the eyes, the brows, etc.

Autologous
Occurring naturally in a certain type of tissue of the body.

Bleaching agents
Slow down or block the production of melanin to lighten age spots and fade areas of hyperpigmentation, e.g. kojic acid, hydroquinone.

Blepharoplasty
Surgery to rejuvenate the upper and/or lower eyelids by removing fatty or excess tissue from the eyelids.

BOTOX
The brand name for Botulinium Toxin, injected into the muscles to smooth out wrinkles by temporarily paralyzing the muscles that cause contraction.

Brow lift
A surgical procedure in which drooping eyebrows are elevated to a higher position.

Cannulae
Long, thin hollow tubular instrument used to extract fat during liposuction.

Carbon dioxide
Laser technology used to resurface facial wrinkles and scars. Can also be used as a cutting tool in surgery.

Cheek augmentation
A procedure designed to give more definition to the cheekbones by implanting artificial materials or grafting bone into the malar region.

Cheek lift
Also referred to as the 'mid-facelift,' this is a surgical procedure designed to lift sagging areas in the mid-face, including around the cheek-bone areas below the eyes.

Chemical peeling
Skin resurfacing, when a chemical solution is applied to the skin so that the top skin layer will peel off.

Chin augmentation
A surgical procedure to build up a recessive chin by inserting a solid silicone rubber implant material or by grafting bone to the chin.

Collagen
Component of human skin that gives it resilience, suppleness and tone. It breaks down with age.

Collagen instant therapy
Injectable purified collagen extracted from cowhide.

Commissure
The area where two anatomic parts meet, as in the corner of the eye or the lips; typically refers to a fold or crease.

Composite lift
An operation designed to lift the skin and underlying soft tissue of the face, brow and upper eyelids; also referred to as the deep plane facelift.

Congenital
Present from birth.

Congenital ptosis
A hereditary condition in which there is a drooping of one or both upper eyelids.

Contraindication
A condition or disease that makes it too risky to perform a treatment or surgery, or to give a medicine.

Corrugator
Muscle that is responsible for causing the glabellar or vertical lines that form between the eyebrows.

Cosmeceutical
A substance that falls between the classification of a drug and a cosmetic, i.e. non-prescription over-the-counter formulations that provide pharmaceutical benefits.

Crow's feet
Wrinkles around the outer corners of the eyes.

Crust
Surface layer formed by the drying of a bodily secretion.

Dermabrasion
A form of skin resurfacing that aims to improve irregular or uneven skin texture and acne scars.

Dermis
The layer of skin composed of collagen and elastin, lying beneath the epidermis (outer layer) and above the subcutaneous layers of skin.

Diode
Contact laser technology that cuts and coagulates tissue.

Dissect
To separate anatomical structures via tearing or cutting through the connective tissue that holds them together.

Drainage
A tube that is inserted in or near a surgical wound to drain excess blood and fluid.

Dry eye
A condition of the eyelids which causes dryness, inflammation, irritation and blurred vision of the eyes caused by low tear production.

Ectropion
A condition of the lower eyelid in which the lid is pulled downwards by the loose eyelid skin or muscles or from having too much skin removed; also called 'lid retraction'.

Embolus
A piece of blood clot, fat or air bubble that breaks away and can infiltrate the bloodstream during surgery.

Endoscopically-assisted surgery

A small, rigid, tube-like instrument called an endoscope is equipped with fiberoptic lighting, which can be introduced into the body through a tiny incision to light up the surgical area shown on a video monitor while the surgeon performs the operation, as in endoscopic browlifting, facelifting, etc.

Entropion

A condition in which the eyelid margin is rolling toward the eye.

Epithelialization

Regeneration of the epithelium or superficial layer of the skin, as occurs after laser resurfacing.

Erythema

Redness of the skin caused by increased blood flow to the area, as in post-laser or other resurfacing treatments.

Excision

Removal via surgical cutting.

Exfoliant

A material that removes dead surface skin cells.

Extrusion

The erosion of skin that causes an implant (chin, lip, breast, etc) to become partially exposed.

Facelift

A surgical operation designed to reposition and support sagging skin and the underlying tissues, and to remove excess skin and fat. Term usually indicates the lifting of the lower two-thirds of the face and neck, but does not include the eyes or the forehead.

Fascia

The sheet of connective tissue that covers the muscles, sometimes used as a graft material.

Free radicals

Destructive form of oxygen generated by each cell in the body that destroys cellular membranes.

Frontalis

The muscle that enables the brows to move up and down, and contributes to the formation of horizontal wrinkles of the forehead.

Genioplasty

To add projection to the chin. The bones are broken so that the chin area can be moved forward and secured in place.

Glabellar

The region between the eyebrows.

Graft

A piece of tissue that is totally removed from one part of the body and transferred to another area of the body.

Haematoma

A localized accumulation of blood in the skin caused by a blood vessel wall rupture; it is a possible complication of surgery and it may have to be drained out.

Hyperpigmentation

An excess of pigment in a skin area causes darkness; can also be caused by sun exposure.

Hypopigmentation

Reduction in the pigment cells in the skin resulting in skin lightening; can occur after resurfacing.

Incision

A cut made into body tissue to perform surgery.

Infection

Collection of bacteria or pus that can occur in a wound.

Intravenous

A tube is inserted into a vein through which medication and fluids are administered, as in anaesthesia.

Jessner's solution

Pronounced 'yes-nerz', a pre-measured solution formulated with Resorcinol, salicylic acid and lactic acid with ethanol, originally developed by Dr Max Jessner at New York University Hospital for the treatment of acne.

Keloid

The overgrowth of fibrous scar tissue.

Laser

Acronym for Light Amplification by the Simulated Emission of Radiation, a device that emits an intense beam that can be precisely directed and controlled.

Lateral hooding

Excess fold of skin between the eyebrow and the outer portion of the upper eyelid.

Lymphatic system

A network of structures, including ducts and nodes, that carry lymph fluid from tissues to the bloodstream.

Laser skin resurfacing

Treatment of skin conditions with a laser, so that a beam of light is focused to penetrate or vaporize tissues. Laser skin resurfacing is used to improve wrinkles, to treat facial veins and to remove sunspots, facial hair, port-wine stains and certain kinds of tattoos.

Lip lift

A surgical procedure designed to create the appearance of larger, more youthful lips, in which a surgeon removes a strip of white skin from around the lip and advances the pink skin into that area.

Liposuction

The removal of fat with a slender hollow instrument called a cannula. This instrument is inserted through a very small incision and attached to a suction machine to vacuum out excessive fat.

Mentoplasty

A shaping or moulding of the chin, such as building up the chin through chin augmentation.

Mid-facelift

Also referred to as a 'cheek lift', this is a surgical procedure to lift sagging areas in the middle face, including around the cheekbone areas below the eyes.

Malar bags

The pouch of loose skin and fluid that sometimes occurs with age below the lower eyelid area.

Malar fat pad

A structure that sits in the second layer of the face below the cheekbone that is frequently re-positioned during facial rejuvenation procedures.

Marionette lines

The vertical creases that form in the corners of the mouth towards the jowls.

Mask lift

A surgical operation in which all of the facial structures, including the deep soft tissues and muscles, are lifted to a depth just above the bone.

Micro-dermabrasion

Mechanical blasting of the face with sterile micro particles that abrade or rub off the top layer of skin, after which the particles and dead cells are vacuumed away.

Milia

Tiny skin cysts that resemble whiteheads; sometimes form after laser resurfacing.

Mid-facelift

Also referred to as a 'cheek lift,' a surgical procedure designed to lift sagging areas in the mid-face, including around the cheekbone areas below the eyes.

Monitoring device

Equipment that is used to closely watch and report the body's vital functions, e.g. heart rate, pulse, etc.

Nasal labial fold

The crease or fold of skin and soft tissues that runs from the outer corners of the base of the nose to the corners of the upper lip.

Necrosis

Dead skin cells.

Neck lift

A surgical operation to lift sagging tissues of the neck and tighten the underlying musculature.

Oedema

Swelling or fluid retention which can occur after surgery or inflammation.

Orbicularis oculi

The muscular body of the eyelid encircling the eye and comprising the palpebral, orbital and lacrimal muscles. The orbital muscle functions to close the eyelids which causes winking or crow's feet.

Outpatient surgery

Ambulatory surgery in which you are discharged later the same day from the recovery room in a hospital, doctor's surgery or clinic.

Phenol

Peeling formula applied to the skin to lighten pigment, soften wrinkles and improve scars; considered to be a deep and more invasive peel.

Photoageing

Skin damage caused by cumulative exposure to the sun's rays, i.e. wrinkles, age spots, fine lines, etc.

Platysmal bands

Vertical strands of the muscle of the neck that can become more prominent with age and are often sutured or tightened during a face- or necklift.

Plication
A surgical technique that involves tucking or pleating.

Procerus
Muscle that works with the corrugator muscles and contributes to the vertical frown lines between the eyebrows.

Ptosis
Pronounced 'toe-sis', a term for drooping as in eyelids, breasts and brows.

Post-operative
After the operation, or after surgery; 'postop'.

Pre-operative
Prior to the operation, or prior to the surgery; 'preop'.

Resect
Removal of a portion of tissue or an organ.

Rhytidectomy
Technical term for a facelift.

Rosacea
A common skin condition of the face that results in redness, pimples, dilated blood vessels and occasional pustules.

Scar treatments
A range of treatments designed to improve the appearance of scars. Among those treatments are surgery and dermabrasion.

Seroma
A collection of clear fluid that may develop following surgery.

SMAS
Acronym for the superficial musculo-aponeurotic system; a layer of tissue that covers the deeper structures in the cheek area and touches the superficial muscle covering the lower face and neck, called the platysma.

Saline
Salt water commonly used as a filler for breast implants and in the course of administering intravenous fluids.

Scleral show
Lower eyelid retraction which exposes the sclera (white part of the eyeball) below the pupil.

Silastic sheeting
Patches or strips of silicone that may be applied to the skin for extended periods to soften and reduce scarring.

Silicone
A synthetic substance used in a gel-like form in breast implants; in a liquid-injectable form for facial areas; and in other medical devices.

Steroids
Any of a large number of hormonal substances with similar basic chemical structure, produced mainly in the adrenal cortex and gonads.

Subcutaneous
Under the skin.

Submental
Referring to the area below the chin.

Subperiosteal
A term for a procedure that goes deep into multiple layers; a lift in which all tissues are separated from the underlying bone structure, thereby considered more invasive, as in brow, face, etc.

Sunblock

A physical sunscreen or barrier against the sun's ultraviolet rays.

Sutures

Strands or fibres used to sew together parts of the body; often referred to as 'stitches'.

Telangiectasia

Small thread veins, as found in the face.

Tissue engineering

The science of production of human tissue ex vivo (outside of the human body), as in growing cartilage in tissue culture.

Tragus

A small extension of the auricular cartilage of the ear, anterior to the external meatus.

Tumescent

A method of anaesthesia where large volumes of local anaesthetic and saline solution are injected to swell the area to be operated on; commonly used in liposuction and body contouring procedures.

Ultrasound

Application of a sound wave, a mechanical vibration of more than 16,000 cycles per second.

Undermining

Surgical separation of tissues from their underlying structures.

UVA

Long wavelengths emitted by the sun which take longer to produce a burn than UVB but penetrate deeper into the skin to cause damage.

UVB

Short wavelengths emitted by the sun that are known to cause premature ageing and skin cancer.

Vector

The direction of pull, as in facelifting, etc.

Vermillion border

The external pinkish-to-red area of the upper and lower lips. It extends from the junction of the lips with surrounding facial skin on the exterior to the labial mucosa within the mouth.

Wavelength

The distance between a given point on one wave cycle and the corresponding point on the next successive wave cycle.

YAG

Abbreviation for yttrium aluminum garnet, a crystal used in some types of lasers.

Index

Acknowledgements

My biggest 'thank you' goes to my family, my daughter Eden Claire, who is wise beyond her tender years, my mother Evelyn, who has the patience of a saint, and Harley, our Lhasa Apso, for putting up with all the late evenings and weekends with me slumped over my keyboard. Also the cracker-jack team of assistants who have helped me juggle it all on both sides of The Pond: Evita, Miriam, Kerry, Vanessa and Anne.

The credit for this volume goes also to the literary professionals at Quadrille, most notably Jane O'Shea and Lisa Pendreigh, and to Anne Furniss for having the foresight to recognize that all women want and need information about aesthetic surgery and cutting edge beauty, even in England.

To my dear friend and colleague Penny Bool, who has made it possible for me to get to know and love London and expand my horizons. No words of thanks would be complete without paying homage to the many incredible and interesting women (and men, too) I have come to know, consulted with, and hopefully guided in their pursuit of excellence in the medical field. You are all the true inspirations for this book.

A final big thank you to Mr Alan Matarasso for having a big heart and generous spirit and for believing in me. Now that the book is written, and I have literally aged 5 years in 2, I'm ready to have my eyes done if you're available.